HOW TO LIVE
TO BE 100
AND ENJOY IT

by STEVEN WEST

in collaboration with

Donald Tyburn-Lombard

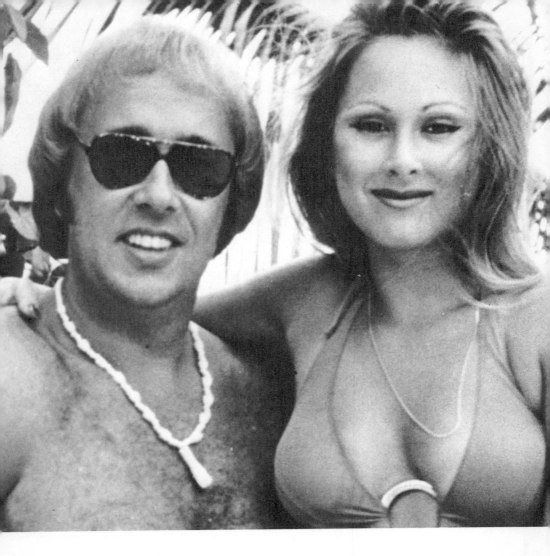

For information, address
Aabbott McDonnell-Winchester Publishers
376 Wyandanch Avenue
North Babylon, New York 11704
(516) 643-3500

ISBN: 0-89519-004-4

To Sherri
May we spend
the next
100 years
together

Written by..Steven West
in collaboration with.............Donald Tyburn-Lombard

Photography by ....Jim Hanson
and Vincient Busby

Research Directors....................................Robert Orgel
....Sandy Brotman
....Beverly Blake

TABLE OF CONTENTS

INTRODUCTION

*Life is an adventure in experience
and when you are no longer greedy
for the last drop of it, it means no
more than that you have set your
face to the day when you shall depart.*

> *DONALD C. PEATTIE*
> *Almanac for Moderns*

This may be the most important book you ever read. It may change your entire outlook on life and aging. Why? Because here, in this book, you will find the equivalent of a real and completely factual Fountain of Youth—a veritable fountain-head of new and startling information concerning your ability to live to 100 years of age and beyond.

Where did this information come from? A thousand different and reliable sources including government agencies, leading scientists and medical investigators; from leading anthropologists and nutritionists as well as from extracts of statistical analysis reports, medical reports and several scientific papers that have been presented to members of the medical and scientific community.

On the other end of the scale, I have also included data from astrological research and psychic investigations.

The sum total of all this information adds up to one simple, inescapable fact: There is every reason to believe that you—regardless of your age right now—are quite capable of living to be 100 years or older. The decision to do so lies in your hands.

Please understand that I am talking about living to that age with full mental, physical and sexual power and vigor. I am talking about living your life to the full extent that you were meant to live; with keen enjoyment of every moment.

I intend to show you tested and practical methods that you can start using right now; simple and effective ways and means that will help you to look and feel years younger and keep feeling that way to 100 years of age and beyond.

I'm going to show you how to protect and expand your mental, physical, sexual and psycho-spiritual vitality so that you will, for the first time in your life, be fully alive, fully aware and capable of enjoying the best that life has to offer.

Long before you are half way through this book you will begin to feel the stirring of excitement and realize that you are fully capable of engaging in a new career, of meeting and enjoying challenging relationships with new and exciting people; of engaging and exploring with uninhibited pleasure all the avenues of sexual delight.

You'll learn new and startling facts about the myths of impotency, frigidity, heredity, radiation, drugs as well as the hidden effects of climate and weather on your actual life expectancy. You'll learn the truth about food, vitamins, cigarettes, coffee and alcohol. That truth will not only set you free, it will add 40, 50, 60 or 70 years to your life expectancy.

If you doubt that living to 100 years of age or beyond is possible—consider the fact that U.S. government figures show barely a million people lived beyond 65 years of age a century ago. Now they estimate that we will have more than thirteen million people, 75 years or older, in the year 2000.

You can be one of them.

The book you are holding will show you exactly how to achieve your goal of a longer, healthier, more vigorous life to 100 years of age and beyond.

Read it—enjoy it—do it!

STEVEN WEST
May 1, 1977
New York, N.Y.

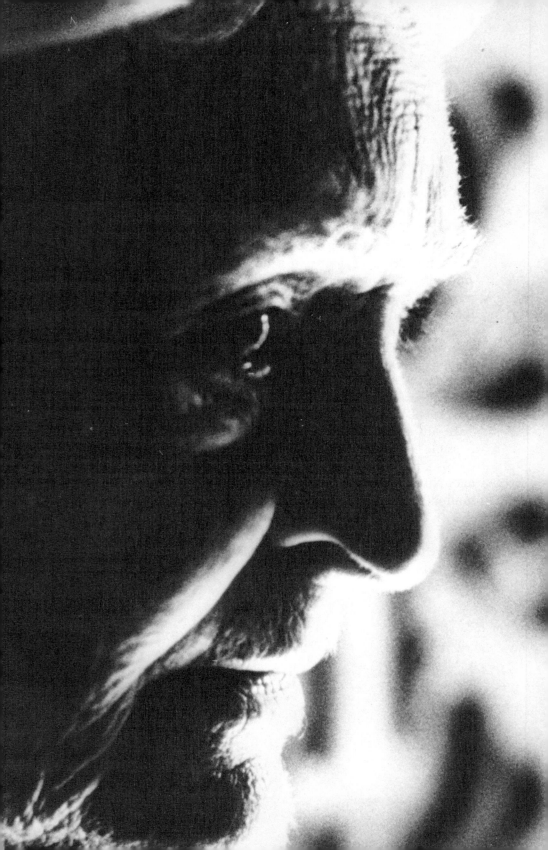

CHAPTER ONE

THE REALITY OF LIVING LONGER

*Every man desires to live long
but no man would be old.*
JONATHAN SWIFT

Let's begin by answering some of the questions that almost everyone asks whenever the subject of longevity is brought into the conversation. Now it's safe to say that virtually everyone has either read or heard about people here and there who have lived beyond 100 years of age. They more or less accept this information at face value (although some people tend to suspect that the birth records were not quite accurate). However much they may believe that it's possible that, on occasion, some men and women do live beyond the age of 100, they sincerely doubt that it can happen to *them*. The questions they then ask follow this sort of pattern:

"But isn't living beyond 100 a kind of freak accident?"

"No, It's neither freakish nor accidental."

"You mean it's a natural thing to live that long?"

"Yes. It's normal and natural."

"For everyone? Not just a select few?

"Every human being on Earth should—barring accidents or natural catastrophe—live to be 125 to 150 years of age."

"I just can't believe that. Look—if that was a fact then millions of people would be living that long—not just a few here and there. Right?"

"Right. Millions of people are living that long—right now."

"I didn't know that."

"You do now."

"All right. Let's say you're right. The total population of the entire world is about four billion people—right?"

"Give or take a little—right."

"Then how come the average life expectancy—on the average is about 70 years of age. I'll even give you 74 years of age in the United States. How come?"

"It's very simple—people really don't want to live that long. The majority of people in the world commit suicide either overtly or covertly."

"I don't understand."

"I mean, very simply, that they either kill themselves consciously and deliberately or they do it subconsciously."

*　　*　　*　　*

And that—in essence—is what this book is all about. I'm going to show you a number of simple ways to stop killing yourself so that you can live to the full life span that you were meant to. I'm also going to show you how to fully enjoy those added years so that you look forward to them—rather than dreading them as you do now.

*　　*　　*　　*

Let's start with some basic facts.

A human being is a mammal. How is the life expectancy of a mammal calculated? The general rule is to multiply by 5, the number of years it takes for the skeleton to fully mature. For example:

DOG: Skeleton maturation 2 to 3 years
Life expectancy—12 to 15 years

HORSE: Skeleton maturation 4 years
Life expectancy—20 to 21 years

MAN: Skeleton maturation 25 to 28 years
Life expectancy—125 to 150 years

THE 3 SHANGRI-LAS

Most people have, at one time or another, read the novel LOST HORIZON by James Hilton. Many have also seen the motion picture. The intriguing factor in the story was the accidental discovery of a hidden valley, high in the Himalayan Mountains, where no one ever aged. There was something in the mineral content of the water—in the type of climate—in the food—that enabled the men and women in this enchanted valley to stay young and vigorous for hundreds of years.

The name of this valley was Shangri-La and it has passed into our language as a synonym for a magical place where men and women stay young and beautiful forever. That concept is just a fairy tale—or is it?

In 1969 The Society of Cardiologists sent a medical expedition to a place called Vilcabamba, in Ecuador, South America. Their purpose was to confirm the reports that most of the men and women lived well beyond 100 and were mentally, physically and sexually active up to the time they died. This medical team made many puzzling discoveries.

Vilcabamba is a hidden valley (the name means 'sacred valley') surrounded by towering mountain peaks. It has been described as 'utterly tranquil'. The temperature, year round is exactly 70° Fahrenheit. Exactly the same amount of sun and rain is received each year. The wind blows from the same direction every day, all year long. The altitude (5000 feet) is quite healthy and because of it there are no mosquitos, spiders or snakes. There is a wide variety of fruit, flowers, vegetables and domestic animals.

There is a total absence of serious ailments, particularly heart disease. In one case, an American suffering from a serious heart ailment, lived in Vilcabamba for a year and experienced a spontaneous improvement in his heart ailment.

Many men and women, well above the age of 100, work side by side with younger people, easily and without fatigue. They live active lives, eat frugally (1,200 calories per day), breathe fresh air and drink sparkling, fresh water from two unpolluted rivers. They have few worries and a keen sense of humor. They enjoy sex just as much at 123 as they did when they were 23.

There is another, high altitude (8,500 feet) hidden valley in the Karakoram Range of the Himalayas. It's called Hunza and it's located in the far, northeast corner of Pakistan. Estimates of the average age according to visiting scientists vary from 95 to 150. There is general agreement that about 50 out of every hundred people in Hunza are over 90. They also agree that at least 6 people in every hundred are over 100 years of age.

Contrast those figures with the United States where 3 people in every 100,000 live to be 100.

Scientists and medical personnel who have been studying the Hunza people are astonished at the mental and physical fitness of the extremely advanced men and women. It is quite common for men over 90 to father children and women 60 years and older give birth to them!

The Hunza people, regardless of age, work hard and play hard. A peculiar form of polo and volley ball are very popular sports with the Hunzukut (the name of the people of Hunza). Again, as in Vilcabamba, the diet is frugal (1,900 calories). Fresh fruit, vegetables, little or no meat, constitutes the main diet. Another peculiarity is the longevity of the fruit trees. In America 25 to 30 years is the average—in Hunza fruit trees continue to grow and bear fruit over 100 years.

The third "Shangri-La" is in the Soviet Union, in a place called Transcaucasia. The population (about 9 million people) has the highest percentage of 100 year old people on Earth. There is no word in their language for 'elderly' or aged—the word they use means 'long centuried.'

In one of the most recent census it was discovered that there were more than 5,000 men and women over 100 years of age in Caucasus. In Abkhazia, there are 15,000 men and women (out of a population of 500,000) well over the age of 90. In further analysis, one of every 300 people in Abkhazia is well over 100 years of age.

Two of the most spectacular (and authenticated) long lives were those of Shirali Mislimov who died at the age of 168 in 1973 and a woman named Tsurba who died at 160. Her case was quite remarkable. At the age of 140 she began to shrink little by little each year and when she died (20 years later) she was only 3 feet tall and slept and died in her crib.

The most astonishing thing about these people is their sparkling good health at advanced ages. Well over 100 years of age and they have their own teeth, good eyesight, beautiful hair and skin and mentally, physically and sexually vigorous.

Here again the diet is frugal (1,700 calories), no alcohol and they do not smoke. They eat fruit and vegetables and get most of their protein from cheeses rather than meat. Clear air, fresh water and an active life are key factors.

Now from these three areas we should be able to extract certain common denominators that will help you to achieve what these people have achieved.

There seems to be one main factor running like a vivid thread through the tapestry of all these lives. *Activity*. These people are constantly active.

They are busy from sunup to sundown with a host of things ranging from work to play. They have a keen sense of humor and they enjoy sex in a hearty, healthy, completely uninhibited manner. They give full range to all five senses. Most of all, they are vividly aware of each other, the world around them, the food they eat, the water and milk they drink and there is an almost total enjoyment of *being*, that seems to permeate their long, fruitful lives.

Another common factor is their diet. Note that in all three cases the caloric intake was low—from 1,200 to 1,900 calories. Contrast that with the average caloric intake of 3,300 calories in these United States.

Now there is something interesting in the *kinds* of foods these long-living people eat. Grain, for example, is a staple in all three 'Shangri-Las'. It's not the same kind of grain that we eat. Ours has been 'refined' which means most of the very important nutrients are discarded and lost. That's why there is so much emphasis on 'adding' vitamins to our grain products. There is something idiotic about removing the natural vitamins and adding artificial ones.

The long-living people use freshly-ground millet and wheat which contains wheat 'germ' the storehouse of a number of vitamins including vitamin "E" which scientists are now beginning to view as the key to sexual vigor and strength.

Another important long-living food is milk and milk products. Particularly the buttermilk, cheese, butter and yogurt these various Shangri-La people make a major part of their diet.

Fruit, of course, is an extremely important factor mainly because of the fructose which provides the only kind of sugar that the human brain can use.

Vegetables are another key factor—not just in themselves but in the way they are eaten. Since, in most areas, there is a lack of ready fuel, cooking is done quickly (if at all) and so none of the vital nutrients are cooked away and lost.

In all three areas, the soil is rich in minerals and the fruit and vegetables grown look beautiful and taste as good as they look. Herbs are an important part of the diet and because there is no need for insecticides (at those high altitudes) vegetables, herbs, lettuce like leaves can all be enjoyed without washing away their natural fragrance and flavor.

Did you notice that meat was, in the main, avoided? Most of these people derive their protein from milk, eggs and cheese rather than meat—more from necessity than preference since there was little meat to be had. Whatever the reason, the fact is that by eliminating meat they eliminated the high amount of saturated fat in their diet. That's the kind of fat that affects the arteries, induces high blood pressure and heart disease.

Scientists, at all three locations, were struck by the extraordinary tranquility of these long-living people. They were calm and relaxed; they worked without undue haste, there was little or no anger or hostility evidenced and—in all—the scientists began to relax and work at a more leisured pace with greater enjoyment.

When we begin to add up all these factors, a pattern begins to emerge that is unmistakable in its implications. Before we verbalize it, let's examine some of the philosophy that is either expressed or implied by these long living people.

Please understand that what I am about to present is a synthesis of the established pattern of thought of a rather large group of people who have demonstrated that they know how to extract the most from life and living.

1. Positive thinking seems to be the prevalent mode. These people simply do not entertain negative thoughts. They think directly, simply and with absolutely no idea that they cannot accomplish what they set out to do.
2. They rarely consider age until it is quite advanced and even then, they do not consider it any reason to stop working, playing or engaging in sexual intercourse.
3. They eat when they are hungry, thoroughly enjoy everything they eat and, in the main, eat sparingly. They are not gluttons simply because there is no need to be. Mentally healthy, physically fulfilled people have no need to use food as a substitute for love—which is the main reason for overweight.
4. The five senses of these people are as keenly honed as a razor. They experience the world around them, the people they live, love and work with, the flowers, the fruit, the vegetables and their handiwork, vividly, intensely and with immense enjoyment. They live to the full potential of their physical and mental capabilities. Sex, to them, is a joyous celebration of love, tenderness, affection and uninhibited sensuality.
5. Breast feeding is a joy rather than a chore. In fact children are treated with respect, admiration and unlimited affection and respond in kind.
6. Crime is literally unthinkable in these communities. That's because there is interpersonal respect that is given and received. Just as there is no breeding ground for mosquitos there is no breeding ground for crime in these real life Shangri-Las.

None of the truly astonishing things we have learned about these long-living people is the result of a fortuitous accident. The established fact that people can live long, fruitful, enjoyable, active lives in peace and harmony has been clearly demonstrated by many scientific investigators.

If this kind of ultimate living had been discovered in only one place in the world then it would have been easy to assume that it was accidental. But it has been found in three different, widely separated places, and, for all we know, may exist elsewhere as well.

The fact is that it has been done, is still being done and will continue to be done by human beings no different than you. Our task is to discover exactly what we have to do to live like that—to enjoy a rich, exciting and fruitful life well past 100.

Obviously we have to consider everything that can affect the length and quality of your life. That means we will have to become conscious of, and pay attention, to everything you eat and drink, the kind of activities you engage in—whether it's work or play—your particular lifestyle, the community you live in, the climate of the area in which you live, the extent and nature of your sex relations, any conditions which may exist that cause stress, tension and anxiety.

We have now presented enough material for you to realize that the answer to the question—"How can I live a longer, more fruitful and more enjoyable life?"—will not be found in a single area, but in many different areas.

It is my intention, in this book, to teach you, step-by-step simple and effective methods of modifying some of your lifelong habits; of adopting new mental attitudes; of becoming a 'friend' to your body; of reaching out and embracing the rich full life that is yours for the taking.

I will need your help and co-operation if we are to succeed. Please keep an open mind and above all trust me. I sincerely want you to reach the goal that we have outlined. I want you to live to the full number of years that you are entitled to. Above all, I don't want them to be empty years. They should be filled with excitement, delight and joy in living—and they can be, if you will be patient and follow the suggestions that I give you as we go along in this book.

Remember what I said, earlier, about people really not wanting to live to an extreme old age? That's the unvarnished truth of the matter. People really do commit suicide, either consciously or unconsciously. New studies by safety authorities reveal that many of the 'accidents' in cars are really disguised attempts at suicide.

Now if you add those figures (which are extremely high) to the number of people who are willfully and deliberately shortening their lives with drugs, alcohol, cigarettes and 'junk' food, then a rather grim picture emerges.

On the other side of the coin there is a brighter and more cheerful aspect. New discoveries by scientists are now being made in foods and nutrients which can help you to look younger and stay younger throughout your life. This is particularly true in the work that is being done with RNA (ribonucleic acid) and DNA (deoxyribonucleic acid). You will learn a great deal more about this in the chapter entitled WHAT YOU EAT IS HOW YOU AGE (Chapter Five).

Right now we will begin to learn about the enemies of long life. Knowledge is power. When you know the enemies that are eating away your life expectancy, you can begin to take steps to overcome them. This is the subject of our next chapter.

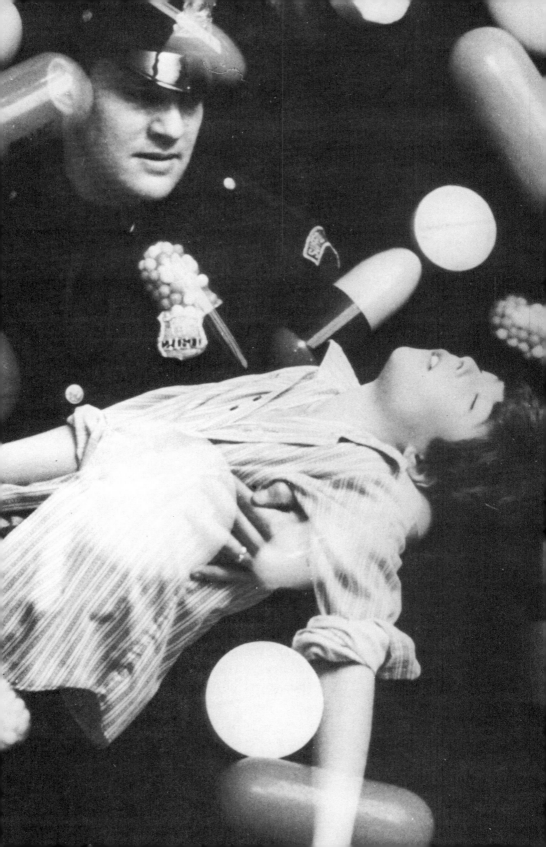

CHAPTER TWO

THE ENEMIES OF LONG LIFE

*We have met the enemy
and they are us.*
POGO

Let's look at some statistical facts and figures. Now I know that this may be distasteful to you but I remind you that you must face the facts of life and death sooner or later. Refusal to face them will not make them go away. One of the things you will learn, as we go along, is that as you become accustomed to facing facts squarely, they will tend to be less of a threat to you. So please bear with me.

We are now going to examine the 15 major causes of death in these United States:

CAUSE Of Death	PERCENTAGE Of Total Deaths
1. HEART DISEASE	37.8
2. CANCER	19.5
3. STROKE	10.2
4. ACCIDENTS	5.3
5. FLU & PNEUMONIA	3.0
6. DIABETES	1.9
7. CIRRHOSIS OF THE LIVER	1.7
8. ARTERIOSCLEROSIS	1.5
9. INFANT MORTALITY	1.4
10. SUICIDE	1.4
11. BRONCHITIS, EMPHYSEMA AND ASTHMA	1.3
12. HOMICIDE	1.1
13. CONGENITAL ANOMALIES	0.7
14. NEPHRITIS & NEPHROSIS	0.4
15. PEPTIC ULCER	0.4

Here's how to read that chart and place it in relation to your life and the life of your friends and relatives. The percentages are based on the figure 100. Can you think of 100 people you know? Then it is safe to say that at least 37 of them have an excellent chance of eventually dying of a heart disease. Those statistics may shock you but it's perfectly true. 37 or 38 people out of each 100 people in these United States will die of a heart attack. 19 out of 100 people will die of cancer and 10 out of 100 will die of stroke.

To look at it another way—you have a 37% chance of dying of a heart disease—a 19% chance of dying of cancer and a 10% chance of dying of stroke.

Yet, with a little care and certain exercises it need never happen to you! You could escape these killers and never be bothered by them for the rest of your life.

The choice is entirely up to you. I'll show you why this is true. Remember what I said about all the things that can affect the length and quality of your life? Well, just by changing a few of those things you can drastically decrease the odds against you and increase the odds for you. In other words, just by adopting a new mental attitude, by engaging in a few simple exercises, and by learning to be a friend to your body, you can increase the possibility of avoiding the three major killers for the rest of your life.

All right. Let's examine some of the killers that we want to avoid. Some of them are visible and some are not.

One of the most dangerous of the invisible killers is *stress*. Stress is a major factor in the three leading causes of death—heart disease, cancer and stroke. Or to put it another way, our lifestyle can produce stress, which in turn leads to the three major causes of death.

Look at the chart below. Do you see that the highest income workers have the highest death rate? At the other end of the scale, the lowest paid workers have the lowest death rate—far below the 'normal' death rate.

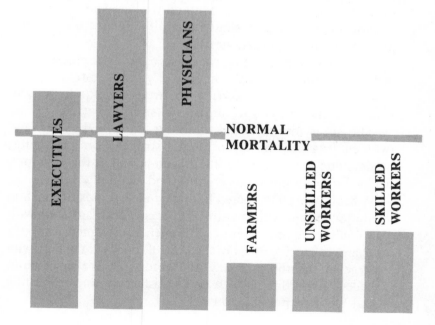

There is a simple, easily understandable explanation for this obvious relationship between high income and a high death rate. It has to do with something called 'environmental stress factors' that are related to high income positions. There are 13.

1. Intense mental effort
2. The pressure of deadlines
3. Lack of physical exercise
4. The strain of updating job-related knowledge
5. The pressure of relentless competition
6. Management use of fear as stimulus
7. Lack of natural air or light during the day
8. Excessive caloric intake at lunch
9. Excessive smoking and coffee drinking
10. Lack of 'finished product' involvement
11. Excessive liquor intake
12. Lack of validation and support
13. Lowered family involvement

These factors have to take a heavy toll in terms of health and in terms of shortened life.

The road to success is not, nor will it ever be, a smooth and serene highway. It's a rocky, pitted, dangerous road that is littered with the wrecks of men and women who have paid a terrible price in terms of shattered health, divorce, alcoholism, drug addiction and early death.

It doesn't *have* to be that way. Success and happiness can be achieved without ruining your health, without destroying your family and without resorting to drugs, tranquilizers and alcohol to permit you to function in stress situations.

The sheer insanity of the lifestyle adopted by men and women engaged in a corporate struggle can be better understood if I said that athletes competing in the Olympics trained on cigarettes, black coffee and alcohol.

A healthy, well tempered body and a clear, positive mental attitude can cope with any stressful, or corporate situation with full confidence and serenity. The men and women who stay cool and calm, regardless of the kind of crisis, are the ones who emerge at the top and stay at the top. They also have an excellent home life as well as a satisfactory and rewarding social life. It is possible to do.

The fact is, no matter what kind of work you engage in; no matter what the corporate situation is, your approach—your mental attitude—your habits—determine exactly how your working hours will affect your life.

You are the one who determines and sets the stage for the relationships you have with people above and below you in your working environment.

You, and only you, are responsible for your attitude towards your job or position. No one makes you bitter, resentful, sullen, suspicious, and morose. These are *your* choices.

I realize that your first instinctive reaction to that statement might be to say, "What am I supposed to do about my negative emotions—suppress them? I can't!"

You're right—you can't suppress most emotions because they're automatic, pre-conditioned responses to certain types of situations. Noticed that I said *pre-conditioned*? That's exactly what your emotional responses are.

You *can* do something about the pre-conditioning. You see, most of the time you are reacting to a previous situation that is similar to the provocative situation. You react without thinking as though you were re-living the original situation.

Here's an example. Suppose, that as a child, you had a deep fear that your father didn't love you as much as your brother or sister. You tried very hard to be good; tried to remember to brush your teeth without being told; tried to remember to comb and brush your hair; tried to remember to sit up straight while eating at the table; tried—in short—to remember and do all the things you were supposed to do.

No matter how hard you tried, sooner or later you slipped and made a mistake and wham! your father would roar like a lion, your heart would jump violently and then you'd be sick to your stomach. Your ears, the tip of your nose and your fingertips would become numb and you'd feel faint.

This reason for that goes back to the beginning of Time, when your ancestors were living a precarious life in a violent and brutal world filled with sudden, unexpected death. To give you a better chance of survival your body developed certain automatic responses. To understand those hair-trigger reflexes, suppose you were flying a twin engine plane at a set speed. Your mind wandered for a few moments and then, suddenly, you realized that you had lost a lot of altitude and were about to crash into a mountain. You jammed both throttles forward and gave the engines a terrific boost of fuel and managed to pull the plane up and over the mountain.

That's exactly what your body does whenever you are faced with sudden fear—or—sudden anger. It shoves the throttles forward and floods your engines with superfuel.

However—it doesn't know whether you are going to *run* (in which case the fuel pours into your legs) or if you are going to stand and fight (in which case it pours into your arms and torso). It simply has to wait and see what happens.

Unfortunately, in our civilized society, we do neither when we receive our shock of fear or anger. We just stand there. So all that fuel pours into our stomach and makes us rather sick.

One trick is—whenever this happens to you—is to tense your arm and torso muscles as hard as you can and then all that package of fuel pours into your muscles and benefits them.

In a moment or two you can relax and you'll feel fine.

Now that takes care of your physiological problem with fear and anger but it doesn't help with your psychological problem. Well, let's see if we can't help there too.

If you can remember to say to yourself: . . .

"This man who is yelling at me is not my father but I am reacting just the way I did when my father yelled at me."

. . . you will shortly be amazed at how calm you can be when you have a crisis with your boss.

In fact, if you can begin to realize that your relations to situations in your home and in your place of business are the result of pre-conditioning as a *child*, you will begin to treat every situation more reasonable and more calmly.

Let me present a typical situation that occurs in business offices all over the world with almost unbelievable regularity. There are two characters in this scene—you may identify with either one of them:

John Doe is a middle management executive who is currently serving what he hopes are his last few months at his present position and salary before being promoted to the first rung of the upper management level.

Mary Jones, his secretary, hopes that when John is promoted, she will go with him as his executive secretary which will place her in a new skill bracket with a higher salary level and regular salary increments.

John is one of 19 Group Leaders in the avionics section of RAD Electronics which is responsible for the total production of technical manuals. John's immediate superior is Robert Coe, the Section Supervisor.

Robert has been mainly responsible for John's rise from writer to editor to assistant Group Leader and finally to Group Leader. He has proposed John for the position of Assistant Supervisor and is keenly concerned with the quality of work from John's department. First because he has to write John's status reports which will, ultimately, have a great deal to do with John's promotion. Second, because as John's sponsor, *Robert's* status report will rise or fall with John's performance. Robert therefore tends to be overly critical and conversely John is highly sensitive to criticism from Robert. In many ways, Robert reminds John of his *father* and he doesn't realize that most of his reaction is pre-conditioned reflex to any situation that is similar to his child-to-father relationship.

Mary likes and admires John but she has a problem whenever situations arise that are similar to situations with her former husband. Her immediate reaction is anger which she tries to suppress (usually with side effects such as loss of efficiency or misplacement of vital papers at critical moments).

Things had been running fairly smoothly until the first official announcement of the opening for assistant supervisor. Technically, all of the Group Leaders were eligible for the position but unofficially it was conceded that John would be chosen. There was little resentment since John actually had both seniority and a superior status record.

Unfortunately John felt a little guilty about his preferred status and began to develop a hypersensitivity about little things that ordinarily wouldn't have bothered him.

He began to pick on little things with Mary; made her do certain documents and letters over when there was no necessity to. Mary tried to overlook this pettiness because she realized the strain and anxiety that John was experiencing. However the more John picked and fretted the more he began to remind Mary of her ex-husband and the angrier she became.

Then, accidentally, she delivered a batch of material directly to the Supervisor without John's usual last-minute check and okay of the material. He was furious when he realized what she'd done and really chewed her out. He coldly reminded her that when he received his promotion he had the final say as to whether she would stay behind or move up with him. That really ticked Mary off but she bit her tongue and suppressed the urge to tell him that it was her high quality work that had contributed to his advancement.

She seethed about it all night and then, in the morning, decided that if he wanted everything letter perfect he would get it that way but it would take a lot longer. Since she was the key factor in the final work, John's department began to fall behind in its daily committments.

John realized that he was being sabotaged but there was nothing he could do about it. He became more and more distracted with his inward raging and extremely resentful of the almost daily chewing out he was receiving from his supervisor. John's previous efficiency began to falter and he began to make little mistakes here and there that grew day by day until finally he made a major goof that placed his Supervisor in a jam with top management.

That did it. John was replaced by another Group Leader and wound up in another section with his title and salary maintained but his future bleak.

Nothing was said to Mary because, outwardly, she had done nothing wrong. But Mary felt terribly guilty for what she'd done to John and shortly afterwards she resigned and took a position with another company.

The sad truth is that none of this needed to happen. It could have been avoided with perception, thought and action on John's part. If he had been able to step back and review the situation calmly and objectively he would have realized that his fears and resentment were out of proportion to the actual situation *now*—and that he was reacting to a situation that he had faced many times as a child.

If he had come to this realization he could have talked it over with Mary, explained what was happening, and enlisted her as a loyal ally instead of turning her into an enemy.

If Mary, for her part, had stopped to realize that the source of her anger was not John's actions but the actions of her former husband, she would have lost the anger and resentment and been able to function efficiently.

The end result of this all-too-common situation in terms of health, for both John and Mary, was quite disastrous. The various kinds of stress contributed to high blood pressure for both of them. It led to improper indigestion, unsettled stomach, headaches, sleepless nights and generally an invitation for one or more physical ailments. It also took years from their life expectancy. Yet, just a little application of common sense, a little perception, a little thought and then positive action, would have cured the situation and healed them.

Empathy (the ability to feel what the other person is feeling and experiencing) is one of the most valuable keys to successful relationships with men or women. Unsuccessful relationships can shorten your life in addition to making you continuously unhappy. Oddly enough, when you stop to think of the other person—when you try to understand their point of view—you stop thinking about yourself and become much calmer and more objective. It's the idea that it is better to give than receive.

Let's see how that might apply to another typical situation.

Again we have two main characters and you can identify with either one of them, if you wish.

Howard is a 'shirt-sleeve' executive, a man who built a small machine shop into a fairly prosperous business. He is now in a position, as head of the company, to put on a tie and jacket and start managing the business from his own office.

He knows that he needs a secretary but dreads the idea of interviewing applicants and hits upon another idea instead. He hires a stenographer from a temporary help agency. The woman they send (Edna) is quite personable, well dressed and highly qualified. After working with her for a week, Howard decides that he'll hire her full time, which is agreeable to Edna.

During the first four months of Edna's employment she was, in all respects, the almost perfect secretary. Howard was well pleased with her, the work went well, and—as he gave her more responsibility—he increased her salary.

Then things began to go wrong, somehow. Little things at first. Howard overlooked them, in the beginning, but then as they grew more consistent, he began to worry about it. It was a subtle thing at first. Their previously cordial relationship began to deteriorate. When he would try to talk to her about the quality of her work he sensed resentment on her part and was hurt and puzzled at her attitude.

It reached the point where Howard began to dread coming into the office because he was certain she'd be tense and cold—or worse than that—on the verge of tears.

He hated the idea of replacing her because he liked her and really didn't want to lose her, but he didn't know what to do. Each time he'd try to approach the situation he only seemed to make it worse. However something had to be done. He knew that without some remedial action the situation would get worse and he just couldn't afford the stress involved.

Howard decided to approach the situation the same way he would tackle a problem in the shop. His first task was to state the problem clearly and in that statement he might find the seed to the solution of the problem. We will call this perception of the problem or a bird's-eye-view of the problem.

1. **Edna was different now than she had been. How?**
   a. Where she had been neat she was now sloppy
   b. Where she had been efficient she was now inefficient
   c. Where she had been cordial she was now sullen
2. **Edna was different (always) (now and then) (certain times)**
   a. Edna was different on Mondays and Fridays
   b. Edna was better on Tuesdays
   c. Edna was her old self on Wednesdays and Thursdays
3. **What did he want?**
   a. He wanted Edna to be the way she was when he first hired her
4. **How can this be accomplished?**
   a. Find out why she's different on Mondays and Fridays and help her to change.
5. **Since the previous attempts to communicate had failed what could he do differently?**
   a. Shock her by telling her that he was about to fire her but wanted to try one more time to see if the situation couldn't be resolved.

That's exactly what Howard did. He brought her into his office on Wednesday (when she seemed almost normal), told her that he was about to fire her unless they could solve the problem of her incredible Monday and Friday behavior.

Edna broke down, cried, and then told Howard the truth about what was happening to her. It seems that her ex-husband had visiting rights with regard to the children and would arrive at dinnertime on Friday night and then stay for the weekend. He would use the children as unconscious hostages to force her to be affectionate with him while they were awake.

When they went to bed he would threaten to make a violent loud scene unless she had sex with him. She had taken to drinking over the weekend to deaden the disgust and repulsion of the virtual rape that she was forced to submit to.

Monday was a very bad day, but by Tuesday she was beginning to pull herself together. Wednesday and Thursday she would work at peak efficiency to try to make up for lost time. Then, on Friday, because she was dreading the thought of going home, she began to fall apart again.

Howard assured Edna it would never happen again. He called his lawyer and the attorney made swift arrangements and Edna's husband, after being informed that he could be arrested and jailed for his actions, ceased to visit after that.

Edna straightened out and became the original efficient and cheerful secretary she had been previously.

Now the point is that this happy result came about because Howard stopped to take time to apply PTA (Perception, Thought and Action). By subjecting the situation to objective analysis, by thinking about exactly what he had to do, he was able to take action and resolve the problem for Edna.

The end result was that two-fold, in that both Howard and Edna's health improved and both of them had a much better chance of living to be 100 years old.

Remember, you always have a choice in life. Nothing is fixed or absolute. If you find yourself in a stress situation that is undermining your health and happiness, don't just suffer it silently and endlessly. *That's slow suicide.* Face it squarely and see if there isn't a solution that can be achieved through PTA (Perception, Thought and Action).

Speaking of suicide, are you aware that many people are unconsciously committing 'slow' suicide every day? Think, for a moment about the people you come in contact with on a daily basis. Think about the people you see at the supermarket or the people you see at work. Do any of them appear to be aging more rapidly than you would expect? Rapid aging (other than the aging that results from severe illness) is usually the outward sign of extreme, self-inflicted mental and physical abuse.

Under normal circumstances you should age quite slowly. Your skin and muscles should stay supple and efficient for 90 to 100 years of age with little wrinkling or sagging. If not then there is either a dietary deficiency or there is a toxic condition caused by the ingestion of cigarettes, alcohol and junk food. Let's take them in order:

CIGARETTES

Now before you wrinkle your nose and say to yourself "He's not going to lecture me about cigarettes—I know all about the Surgeon-General's report. I know all about how bad cigarettes are for my health. It's not going to make a bit of difference *what* he says about them—I'm going to go right on smoking."

If that's the way you feel—okay. It's your life. But please believe me when I say that you are wrong when you say that you know all about the dangers of cigarettes. You don't know the half of it or you wouldn't still be smoking.

Think about it this way, for the moment. Suppose that I told you that for eight hours each day I was not going to permit you to breathe fresh air? Worse than that, I was going to force you to breathe poisonous gases that would shorten your life and undoubtedly cause heart disease or cancer.

You'd consider me a cruel and inhuman monster, wouldn't you? Not that I could blame you for thinking that. But isn't that exactly what you do when you insist on chain smoking? Who is being inhuman then?

You're only given one body during your lifetime. It's about the finest creation in the universe. With proper care and just minimum maintenance it can last about 150 years.

You're shaking your head. You're arguing that you do not chain-smoke. You only smoke in moderation, is that it? In other words you only inhale poison gas occasionally? Is that what you're saying? Well, let's see where that puts you.

According to the best medical evidence the two major causes of death are heart disease and cancer. Almost 58% of all death can be traced directly to these two killers. Cigarette smoking has a direct link to both of them. Here's how:

People who smoke one pack of cigarettes a day have 8 times the chance to have lung cancer than non-smokers. People who smoke 1 to 2 packs per day are 18 times more susceptible to cancer of the lung and 2 to 3 packs make it 21 times more.

Still think that smoking in moderation is safe? Then listen to these figures and tell me how safe it is.

1. Emphysema (another killer) is directly linked to smoking
2. Smokers have a greater chance of dying between the ages of 35 and 55 than non-smokers. Three to four times more!
3. Coronary heart disease strikes 50% more men who smoke than those who don't smoke.
4. The death rate from coronary heart disease is 70% higher in cigarette smokers than non-smokers.

I could go on with statistics and still not really impress you with the seriousness of tobacco addiciton (which is what it amounts to) but maybe the Surgeon General's Report on Smoking would give you deeper insight. It's available (free of charge) from the U.S. Government Printing Office, Washington, D.C. Write for it. You will really be amazed at the facts it offers.

Here's something else to ponder. Since the facts about the dangers of smoking have been published all over the world, smoking has *increased* rather than decreased!

In the United States smokers spend close to 9 billion dollars a year. In the Soviet Union the figure is close to 3 billion dollars. In some countries, the tobacco industry is a state monopoly. In Italy, for example, the government makes a gross *profit* of 2 billion dollars; in Spain it's $210 million; in Switzerland it's $60 million; in Norway it's $70 million and in Sweden $350 million.

There's a lot of profit in tobacco addiction. That's one of the reasons why the tobacco industry in these United States *spends* more than $300 million dollars in advertising each year. They want you to go on smoking regardless of whether or not it kills you. That's why you see magnificent, full color magazine ads with handsome men and beautiful women either smiling with deep sincerity or apparently achieving an orgasm with each drag on the particular cigarette.

The subtle suggestion is that you can be rugged, loaded with machismo and sex appeal just by smoking (cowboy ads) or sophisticated and successful (man about town ads) or possibly terrible erudite and deep into research (graduate college type ads). That's the *male* appeal.

With women it ranges from the long legged, slinky type *(you've come a long way, baby)* to the open man's shirt, outgirl type who looks at you with sincere eyes and a faint smile on her tanned and healthy face and tells you that *"now you can have taste and low tar"* (this is the so called 'honest approach') and then you have the flat out 'comparison' ads which list every cigarette made (their cigarette is in bold face type) showing the lowest tar and nicotine content.

Madison Avenue is out to get you to smoke—and they are succeeding. There is more cigarette smoking going on now than at any time in our country's history. During the time from the original issue of the Surgeon General's report to now—per-capita cigarette smoking has more than doubled!

Do you begin to get the feeling that just about everyone has decided to commit suicide? Based on the unmistakable evidence that has been submitted by every medical and scientific authority that cigarette smoking is a definite link to heart disease and cancer you *know* that smoking will kill you.

If we concede that the majority of Americans (as well as people in other countries) are moderately intelligent then the only answer has to be *deliberate* suicide. It has to be.

Now since you are reading a book on how to live to be 100 years old or better, I can only assume that you have a serious interest in attaining that goal.

Then may I make a suggestion? If you are still smoking please stop. I mean that seriously. *Stop killing yourself.* Let me make a further suggestion. Are you smoking right now, while you're reading this book? Then get up—go to the kitchen—and pour yourself a glass of milk or water.

Bring it back and put away the cigarettes. Each time you feel that you want a cigarette—take a sip of water or milk. I assure you the urge will be immediately satisfied. It's a psychological trick that will help you to cut down on your cigarette smoking almost immediately and eventually eliminate it altogether.

Here's another excellent way to begin to eliminate this killer habit. Place your pack of cigarettes in a plastic bag then fold the bag over several times and put a rubber band around it. When you want a cigarette you will have to take the time to open the bag. This will make you aware that you are about to smoke another cigarette. It will give you time to make a decision. If you decide to skip the cigarette until the next time you have the urge you will immediately begin to cut your smoking in half.

You see, with most smokers, they have the cigarette in their mouth *automatically* without being aware that they have it.

The pack is usually right at hand. They extract and light a cigarette and start smoking without even realizing that they have. When they have to take time to unwrap the plastic they become conscious of what they're doing and that, oddly enough, is half the battle. Try it. You have a lot to gain (like added years) and absolutely nothing to lose.

A friend of mine who was a real addict (five packs a day!) tried an interesting experiment. He decided to give up smoking for just 24 hours. He began his no-smoking period at 10:00 p.m. (as he went to bed) because he reasoned that this gave him a start of 8 hours on his 24-hour project.

The next morning he reminded himself of the 8-hour gain and decided to see if he could add another eight hours without smoking. That would bring him to 2:00 p.m.

When he looked at the clock at 2:00 p.m. he reminded himself that he had now gone 16 hours without smoking. If he could only hold out until bed time (another 8-hour stretch), he knew he would have it made because he would have reached his 24 hour period. Then he realized that all he had to do was go to sleep and in the morning he would have stretched it to 32 hours!

When he awoke the following morning he was so elated that he decided to try for just one more period of 8 hours. Just until 2:00 p.m. which would mean a stretch of 40 hours. That would have been the longest he'd ever gone without smoking. He made it until 2:00 p.m. and it really wasn't difficult. In fact, he realized that if he could make it to bed time he'd not only have totalled up 48 hours but with the 8 hours sleep time he could bring it up to 56 hours.

My friend is still adding up the hours—8 hours at a time and now when you ask him how long it's been since he had a cigarette he usually glances at his watch and then announces something like, "Four thousand, seven hundred and fifty six hours and 12 minutes."

But he still does it in 8 hour stretches.

I should also add that he looks ten years younger, can keep up with youngsters in a stiff game of tennis and is one of the happiest men I know.

Would you like to try for your first 8 hour stretch tonight and see how far you can go? I can guarantee that it will put new life in your tennis game, in your work and in your bedroom playground wherever it is.

ALCOHOL

An item you might find interesting is this statistic: Americans spend more money for liquor per year ($15 billion) than they do for education, medical expenses and religion *combined*! The breakdown is interesting:

1. *Distilled Spirits* (Whiskey, Vodka, Gin, etc.)
   750 million gallons
2. *Beer* (Domestic and Imported)
   100 million barrels
   6 *billion* cans
3. *Wine* (Domestic and Imported)
   250 million gallons
4. *Moonshine* (Illegal Whiskey)
   125 million gallons

Let's say that Americans drink approximately 2 billion gallons of alcohol each year. Drinkers usually smoke so in addition we can add the 544 billion cigarettes they smoke at the same time. It's a pretty combination.

Is it any wonder that 67% of Americans are killed early by heart disease, cancer and stroke between the ages of 35 and 55? The only wonder is that there aren't more deaths.

You mean you didn't know the truth about alcohol? You thought that alcohol in moderation had some beneficial effects? Wrong. *Dead wrong.* Alcohol is pure poison. It's also a rotten tranquilizer because it gives you a brief lift and then drops you like a stone to a depression that was worse than the one you started with.

Alcohol is also an *impersonal* people killer. It kills the sober as well as the drunk. According to the American Safety Council an average of 30,000 men, women and children are killed in alcohol-related accidents on our streets and highways. That's the equivalent of wiping out an entire city of 30,000 people each year! That's only part of the story, however.

How outraged would you be if you read a headline news story that a homicidal maniac had entered a large American city and slashed, maimed and crippled every man, woman and child—the entire population of 500,000 residents?

That's the annual toll produced by alcohol related auto and pedestrian accidents in these United States.

The tragic part is that most of the deaths and most of the crippled victims are innocent victims who were sober!

Here's another grim pair of statistics. Half of the murders and one third of the suicides in this country are directly related to alcohol. Incidentally, there has been new thinking about single driver (alcohol-related) accidents which may be *concealed* suicides (for insurance purposes).

In addition to all that, there is the fact that many accidents and injuries in the home are also alcohol-related. Accidental drowning, falls, fire-related deaths, the battered wife and the battered child are also alcohol-related.

Accidental food inhalation is the sixth leading cause of accidental death in the United States. The culprit—alcohol.

Do you still think that alcohol is a simple, harmless social libation? Are you still secure in your casual statements that, "One or two drinks never hurt anyone." or—"A little drinking is good for you. It aids digestion and it keeps your arteries supple." or—"As long as you drink in *moderation* it's all right." Does that sum up your attitude towards alcohol?

Would you care to repeat those statements to a shattered survivor of an alcohol-related car crash which has just killed his wife, mother and two small children?

What do you think when you read about a drunken driver that has managed to involve two or three cars in a terrible smashup that wipes out entire families?

Do you shake your head and say, "People like that just horrify me. They shouldn't be allowed to drive. They should take their license away permanently."

You, of course, would never do anything like that. You would never drive while you were 'under the influence'—would you? Are you sure? Would you like to take a quiz?

TRUE or FALSE?

1. I sometimes take a drink or two to help me sleep _____
2. I don't like liquor but I'll take a drink to relax _____
3. I'm more comfortable with people who drink ____
4. Everybody knows how well I 'hold' my liquor _____
5. It's all right to have wine with your dinner _____
6. Even if you don't want another drink, it's only polite to let your host or hostess 'freshen' your drink _____

Score yourself 10 for each true answer and 5 for each false answer. Be honest with your answers or you won't learn anything about yourself. 35 or more is a danger sign.

You might be interested to know that the majority of people answer TRUE to most of those statements. That helps to explain why Americans consume so much liquor.

There's another reason. It has to do with good old Madison Avenue—the boulevard of ambiguity and promises.

Their superb blend of great photography and creative copywriting manages to impart a highly acceptable aura to this legally poisonous drug which mains, cripples and kills battalions of innocent men, women and children each year. I offer samples of the advertising copywriters art which I have coupled with appropriate headlines.

For a Tequila Advertisement:

> When you raise your glass
> you'll raise a few eyebrows...
> but you've done that before!

Newspaper Headline:
DEATH PLUNGE CAR RAISED FROM RIVER

For a famous Scotch Advertisement

> What better way to ring in the holidays
> and express the spirit of friendship?

Newspaper Headline:
PREDICT RECORD HOLIDAY DEATH TOLL

For a drink you have with beer:

> Use two hands! For a feeling
> as pleasant as a Danish sunset!

Newspaper Headline:
SUNSET BOULEVARD CAR CRASH KILLS SIX

For a Dry Sherry Advertisement:

> The drink that's light enough
> to fit into a heavy afternoon.

Newspaper Headline:
FIVE DEAD IN AFTERNOON RUSH HOUR PILE UP

For an Italian Liqueur:

> A potion of love with a provocative
> bouquet. Try it tonight.

Newspaper Headline:
DRUNK DRIVER KILLS FAMILY OF FOUR

The siren song that Madison Avenue sings about alcohol is so patently absurd and improbable that you wonder why the usually alert FTC (Federal Trade Commission) doesn't do something about it. They promise—which is loud and clear—states that liquor will make you friendlier, sexier and, above all, happy and successful. Let's examine each promise:

1. FRIENDLIER
> More physical violence in the home, in the streets, in restaurants and bars is directly related to drinking than to any other factor. **Friendlier is OUT.**

2. SEXIER
> Impotence in men and frigidity in women can be directly related to drinking. **Sexier is OUT.**

3. HAPPIER
> Alcohol gives you a brief lift and then drops you like a stone and you're unhappier than ever. Without a doubt **Happier is definitely OUT.**

4. SUCCESS
> When American industry admits that one of its biggest problems is keeping executive on the wagon and failing, then **Success is OUT.**

All right. Let's forget about the Madison Avenue hogwash. What about the physical effects of alcohol on your body? Or are you like the lady who smiles and says, *"I'm all right because I never drink hard liquor—just beer."* She then looks around, leans over and says, quietly and confidently, *"Beer is really a nutritious beverage, you know."*

Really? When a 16-ounce can contains as much alcohol as a 1½ ounce shotglass of 100 proof whiskey?

"I don't believe in drinking," a friend remarked recently, *"but I think it's only civilized to have wine when I dine."* He didn't believe me when I told him that a dainty 3½ ounce wine glass contained as much alcohol as a ½-ounce shot glass filled with 100 proof whiskey.

"I may have a few scotch highballs, just to unwind," a lovely lady remarked to me and then added, *"but I lace them liberally with soda to dilute the liquor."* She was shocked to learn that the soda's carbonation helped her to absorb the alcohol at a faster rate which meant she got 'high' quicker.

The fact is, that until quite recently, physicians would, on occasion, recommend a 'little port' or a little wine to some patients on the general assumption that since alcohol dilates the blood vessels in the skin and increases cutaneous circulation it might also increase arterial circulation and thus be beneficial to the patient.

The truth is that alcohol actually decreases arterial circulation and can help create hardening of the arteries. Since hardening of the arteries is a disease associated with aging (an early death) it might be wise for anyone with a desire to live to be a hundred years of age or better—to take the time to consider whether they wish to continue to drink. It's your choice. No one can make the decision for you. If you want to take the chance—go right ahead. Just realize that the odds against you grow with each drink you take.

That brings us to one of the number one problems in this (and other) country. That's the 'alcoholic'—the real honest-to-goodness *addict*. That's what an alcoholic really is, a drug addict. His drug happens to be alcohol. But it all adds up to the same thing. Your real alcoholic is just as afraid of the pain of withdrawal as your heroin addict.

The big difference is that a heroin addict knows that he's an addict. He is bitterly aware of it every time he needs a 'fix' which is both illegal and terribly expensive.

To show you what the difference is just consider that the alcohol addict can buy a 'fix'—an *ounce* of liquor—for about $1.00 to $1.50 whereas a heroin addict has to pay a street price of $30.00 to $90.00 for a *grain* of heroin. There are 437 grains in an ounce.

If your alcohol addict had to pay $30.00 to $90.00 for a shot of liquor he'd realize that he was an addict in a hurry rather than deluding himself or herself about being a 'social' drinker.

The fact of the matter is that the alcoholics are all over the land as thick as the sands of the sea. From the rich and famous to the poor and anonymous, the addiction is exactly the same. Recently we have heard from more famous 'cured' alcoholics than at any other time in our history. The famous alcoholics cover the entire spectrum of American life—politics, show business, law, science, medicine, religion, the military, no area is immune. You can be certain that you will hear more and more about the mounting problem of alcohol addiction in the years to come. But what about right now. What about *you?*

Are you an alcoholic? Don't shake your head. How do you know whether you are or not? Want to find out, right now? Take the quiz honestly. Answer the questions truthfully. Just remember if you aren't honest with yourself, *you* are the loser. If you catch alcoholism addiction early, it can be cured. If you wait too long it can wreck your life and eventually kill you.

Take the test now and find out once and for all if your suspicions about yourself are correct or not. Look—there isn't a drinker alive who hasn't asked that question mentally. Now you have a chance to find out—all by yourself.

YES or NO

1. Do you actually know how much you drink? _____
2. Do you occasionally minimize how much you've had? _____
3. Do you drink faster in the beginning to get a quick 'high'? _____
4. When you're very tired do you have a 'pick-me-up'? _____
5. Ever have a drink just to chase away the 'blues'' _____
6. Does drinking make it easier to cope with worry? _____
7. Do you stop for a 'quick one' before going home? _____
8. Do you have a drink in the bar car on your commuter train? _____
9. The morning after a heavy party do you forget what happened? _____
10. Have you ever lost time at work because of severe hangovers? _____
11. Do you drink by yourself when you're home alone? _____
12. Do you look forward to a drink right after work? _____
13. When you come home after work are you ready for a drink? _____
14. Are you pleased if a drink's waiting for you when you get home? _____
15. Are you friendlier after you've had 'one or two'? _____
16. Do you think you can 'hold your liquor' better than most people? _____
17. Have you ever thought about giving up liquor for good? _____
18. Do you know how much you spend on liquor and/or beer per week? _____
19. Do you know how many cans of beer you've had in the last month? _____

Add up your total number of YES answers. Now remember that you promised to be honest in this quiz. Were you? Did you really answer every question with complete candor? If you did, then you already know the answer to your question. You don't need me to tell you whether you're in trouble or not. How many YES answers did you have? 3 - 5 - 6? The fact of the matter is if you answered any one of the questions 1 through 17 with a YES, you're in trouble. If you answered the last two with NO you're also in trouble. You'd better take a good hard look at your drinking, right now and make a decision. If you can't stop drinking for good—then get help.

First get a complete checkup from your family physician and find out exactly what kind of shape you're in. Next, look up Alcoholics Anonymous or the National Council on Alcoholism in your local phone book. There's plenty of help out there if you really want to be helped. If you don't want help and you don't want to stop drinking, *then think about that attitude*. Are you intent upon committing suicide—the slow hard way? That's what most alcoholics are doing, you know.

Maybe what you need is therapy—that's available, too. Many large companies now offer psychiatric help as part of their benefit package. Find out about it. There's no stigma attached to it. No more than there is to pneumonia or flu. It's just another disease and can be treated.

The point is, for the sake of your family, if not for yourself, you should do something about it—now.

In our next chapter we're going to take you on a guided tour of your body and make you familiar with how it works and how to keep it in good working order.

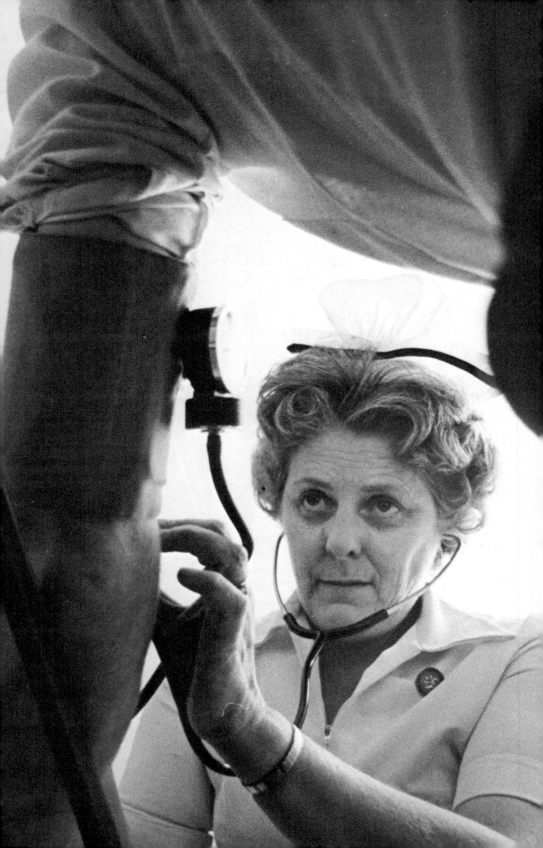

CHAPTER THREE
LEARNING ABOUT YOUR BODY

*No knowledge can be more satisfactory
to a man than that of his own frame, its
parts, their functions and actions.*
                    THOMAS JEFFERSON

Did you ever notice the strange fact that you are never aware of your body when you're well and happy? The only time you really think about your body is when you're sick or injured and then you are deeply concerned—but aware of your abysmal ignorance of what makes your body tick. You suddenly become very dependent upon your family doctor and watch him anxiously while he pokes, pries, weighs and measures and fusses about you liike a mechanic with a rare vintage car who wonders whether he should bother restoring it or not.

That's when you tell yourself that, by golly—*as soon as you're well you're going to take the time to find out about your body*. But you get well and forget all about it—until the next time it happens—and then you make the promise all over again. Well, relax—you are about to take a guided tour of your body in plain, everyday language without a single Latin quotation to make you think your guide is really erudite.

I would like to start with a simple way to make you begin to appreciate what a fantastic creation your body really is. If you were going to buy a new car, for example, you would read about it—find out what kind of mileage it offered, how good a repair record it has, what kind of options and accessories were available—and, in general, become pretty knowledgeable before you spent your hard earned thousands of dollars.

Yet, here you are, with a mechanism that you couldn't buy for a billion dollars (I know a couple of billionaires who tried) and all you know about it is that you have to feed and water it, wash it, clothe it and occasionally rest it. That's about it—except that if you damage it—it bleeds. Then you put a bandaid on it and forget it.

If you will bear with me, perhaps I can generate a little enthusiasm for the incredible mechanism you are lucky enough to own. We'll start with the basic idea of what your body is.

Your body is a totally automated, electro-chemical factory. It's designed to operate continuously without any direction or instructions from you at all. Your only obligation is to supply it with raw materials like food and water. The better the quality of the food and water, the better the quality of the many products your factory will produce. With a little thought and simple care, you can keep this factory going at full capacity for about 125 years, give or take a decade.

Now about the products that your factory produces; there are quite a few of them and—in the main—no one has ever found a way to produce them cheaper, quicker or better.

Take blood manufacturing, for example. Your blood producing plant is in the marrow of your bones. This handy little section produces and maintains about 6 quarts of blood in your body. The amount of blood in any human body is usually between 1/20 to 1/13 of the total weight of the body. The more fatty tissue you carry around the more blood is required and the harder your pumping station (your heart) has to work.

We're going to have a lot to say about your heart later on, but right now, let's stick to the subject of blood, which is really quite interesting. Your blood is a fantastic conveyor belt which does double duty at astonishing speed. In 15 seconds, about 24 billion blood cells have flashed around your entire body in an amazing pickup and delivery service. Your blood not only delivers fresh oxygen and nutrients but it also picks up the garbage at the same time. It's quite a stunt that requires precision of a degree of nicety that no scientist would dare to try to imitate with the biggest and most sophisticated computer.

It means that every single cell in your body has been fed, aired, repaired and cleaned in 15 seconds by this miraculous conveyor belt. Oxygen is one of the most important ingredients. Without the constant supply, the cells die— immediately. There is no delay—no reprieve—the death of the cells is instantaneous.

Now, perhaps you can appreciate what happens with every puff you take on that cigarette. Billions of cells do not receive their supply of oxygen—and they die. Billions of cells are not repaired in time—so *organs* begin to falter. When enough organs falter—the entire body dies. It's that simple.

Now exactly what is this amazing substance called blood? You should think of it as a rapidly moving stream of fluid— which is called plasma—that carries a number of special microscopic machines along with it. Plasma is mostly water (about 90%) about 9% protein and about 0.9% salts. There are traces of sugar, urea, uric acid and other things.

The most important part, of course, are the machines called corpuscles. There are red corpuscles and white corpuscles. The red corpuscles are mainly oxygen carriers. There are about 5,000,000,000 red corpuscles in each cubic centimeter of blood. That's a lot of little machines but, as you can appreciate, you have to have a lot if you're going to carry oxygen to every cell in your body in 15 seconds.

The white corpuscles are something special. There are only about 11,000 white corpuscles per cubic millimeter of blood. That means there are 400 to 500 red corpuscles to each white corpuscle. But the white corpuscles are mighty important. There are five different kinds. Each does a different job when it reaches the cell. Unlike the red corpuscles which just deliver oxygen and pick up carbonic acid gas for the return trip to the lung exchange center, the white corpuscles are a combination disposal, repair, rebuilding and death squad. All foreign bacteria and micro-organisms are killed and eaten on the spot. New tissues and walls are built, erected and nailed down and the cell is cleaned and tidied up in that 15 second flash around the entire body. Here again, if we've been introducing all sorts of poison like alcohol, cigarettes and junk food, the white cells are in short supply so a lot of the important action doesn't happen when it should—and disease begins to run rampant.

Now let's talk about the pumping station—the heart—which is a really incredible machine that pumps (beats) about 150,000 times in a 24 hour period—keeps pumping without stopping for up to 125 years if its kept in good repair.

In that same period, the amount of blood that passes through the heart (every 24 hours) is the equivalent of 10,000 quarts of blood. Just imagine lining up 10,000 quarts of milk and you can get an idea of how much this represents in sheer volume. The blood in your body makes about 5,000 round trips every 24 hours! In just 50 years your heart will pump the equivalent of 45 million gallons of blood through your body without stopping.

Now the interesting thing about your heart is that it's like the engine room in a ship. When the captain calls for more power he calls for full speed ahead. When your body activity speeds up, your heart has to deliver more oxygen and has to pump blood faster. It can deliver tremendous bursts of power under emergency conditions—if it's in good shape. Now all demands on your heart are not just from physical exertion—eating places a greater demand—and overeating places an emergency demand on the heart. If you make too many emergency demands when your heart is weakened by disease or improper conditioning—the pump fails—and you die. It's that simple.

One of the most important (and the largest) gland in your body is rarely talked about. That's the liver. It generally makes up about a fortieth of your weight. In other words if you are a woman weighing 120 pounds, it's a safe bet that your liver weighs about 2½ pounds. A 160 pound man carries around a 4 pound liver. So it's big—and it's important—so why don't you hear more about it?

Mainly because your liver has an amazing ability to heal and reconstruct itself in spite of terrible punishment. And it is punished with all sorts of poisons (drugs, alcohol, starches, concentrated proteins) introduced through improper diets, debauchery, and plain stupidity.

Most people think that cirrhosis of the liver (7th leading cause of death in these United States) is a disease of alcoholics exclusively. Wrong. People who try to live on an exclusive sandwich diet can wind up with cirrhosis of the liver. The reason is excessive *starch*. Keep pounding starch molecules into your liver and it will curl up and die—and you with it. A heavy diet of meat (which is murder on the liver when ingested as a steady diet) will give you an inflamed liver in short order. It's easy to spot people with bad livers—they're so tired all the time they can hardly get out of their own way. They're foot draggers because it's such an effort to lift their feet. They also have terrible posture.

All they have to do, to spring back to life, is give their liver a rest—just by eliminating meat, starches and cooked fats—and their livers will come back to life like a miracle. So will they. It's like a new lease on life.

You see, just about everything you put in your mouth, whether it's solid or liquid, winds up in the liver for special processing. In addition to eliminating any poisonous elements, the liver transforms the material into specialized repair items which the blood then carries to the cells on its 15 second reconstruction tour of the body.

There are certain juices left over which go to the gall bladder (mostly as bile) which uses them in the digestive process.

Let's move on, now, to one of the most important systems in our body—the kidney system. We have two kidneys, which gives you an idea of how important they are. You see, next to oxygen, pure water is the most necessary item on your menu. You may not have thought about it (unless marooned in a desert for several days without water) but you can die very quickly without water. It's strange, but you could last about a month without food, but less than a week without water would absolutely destroy your body beyond redemption. You have to consider that water is like the electrolyte in your car battery. If your battery fluid goes below a certain level you wind up with 'dead cells' and a dead battery. Same thing with your body. If your body fluids drop below a certain level you wind up with a lot of dead cells and eventually a dead body.

Where do you get your water? Not just from the tap, but in coffee, tea and milk—in fruit juices and vegetables. Now getting most of your water from coffee, tea or milk isn't the greatest idea in the world because of the added ingredients. I don't have to tell you that coffee and tea has poisonous substances. (I use the word poisonous to mean any item that doesn't help your body—but only puts a burden on it.) However, you may not be aware that too much milk isn't helpful either. Now please understand that when I refer to 'milk' I'm really talking about the ridiculous substance that passes for milk in our society. It has about as much resemblance to real milk as a Volkswagen has to a Mercedes. If you have ever lived on a farm you know what real milk is.

There are a couple of valid reasons for cutting down on your milk drinking. One is the fact that many of the benefits that milk used to offer (enzymes, anti-bodies and natural hormones) are destroyed by pasteurization. So is the calcium which is one of the main reasons why we are told that children should have lots of milk. Another disturbing thing about milk, of late, is the fact that the artificial additives and chemicals that a cow ingests with its food, eventually goes into the milk that we drink. Think about that, the next time you decide you want a nice, cool drink of milk. Try a glass of water instead.

Anyway, once water (in whatever form) arrives in your body, it enters the bloodstream and winds up in your kidneys where about 30 billion cells filter out the impurities. Your kidneys handle about 4½ gallons of water a day with ease. Remember that 15 second flash around your body that your blood stream makes? Well it flashes through your kidneys on the way. Kidney filtering goes on all the time. About 2 to 2½ pints of water go to your bladder for elimination. Excess water is usually stored in your muscles and liver.

That's why people who go on insane crash diets get the idea they're losing weight fast. They're not—they're losing stored up water excess.

The next time you are about to order that sixth cup of coffee—stop—think about your poor overworked kidneys and take a drink of water instead.

Moving right along, on our guided tour, we now arrive at a part of the plant known as the air/oxygen intake section commonly called the lungs. They're a spongy-looking mass of little cells in bunches (about 400 million of them) which can separate oxygen from each pint of air they take in. When the lungs exhale, they expel millions of molecules of carbonic-acid gas. It's a two stroke system. Oxygen on the in-stroke, carbonic-acid gas on the out-stroke. Works beautifully unless you smoke. Then there's bad news because the tar begins to build up on the cells and prevents the cells from carrying on the oxygen separation. When the tar builds up to a high enough irritant factor, you will find that you have an almost constant cough. The cough is a reminder from your lungs that things are really getting a bit congested and could you ease up and cut out smoking for awhile? But you pay no attention to the signals—just go on smoking and coughing—right up to the point where you won't have breath enough to cough. Then you'll stop coughing—for good.

Incidentally, even non-smokers can louse up their lungs by drinking too much milk and eating too many starchy foods. That puts a heavy coating of mucous on the lungs and leads to a lot of racking coughing. Just ignore the coughing, keep drinking milk heavily and eating starchy foods and you're bound to wind up just like your friend the smoker—without a cough left.

Why am I being so tough about this? Because I really would like to see you start to enjoy your life—and have enough time left to enjoy it. That's all. It really hurts me to see so many people—of every age—just wrecking their bodies and their life expectancy for something they don't even enjoy.

Now don't tell me you enjoy smoking. Maybe the first puff, but all the rest is purely automatic. Half the time you don't even know that you're smoking—so how much enjoyment is there?

Want to smoke the heavy smokers in any crowd? Easy—just follow the coughs. If you really want to shock a heavy smoker, get a tape recorder and tape his coughs in any one-hour period. He has no idea that he coughs that much. He's so used to it that he hardly hears it anymore.

Now we come to a subject that may be a bit distasteful to you but it's terribly important—so please bear with me. I promise I'll be brief.

One of the factors most critical to good health (and long life) is the proper and regular elimination of waste products from the body. In addition to being important, elimination is one of the most dangerous of all the bodily processes.

To understand why it's so dangerous, we have to start at the beginning, when you first place food in your mouth. Your mouth is really a pre-processing station and the longer food stays in your mouth and is chewed before swallowing, the better your health will be. You see, food that isn't chewed enough or pre-digested by the enzymes in your saliva, is just not being properly digested in your stomach (if at all).

While you're chewing your food, your stomach is making all kinds of preparations. It's secreting gastric juices (mostly a form of hydrochloric acid), so that when the pre-digested food arrives, it can be broken down easily into chemically treated particles that can be absorbed by the small intestine.

Now most of the liquid that you drink, as you eat, is quickly absorbed through the walls of the stomach. So is most of the liquid that your stomach squeezes out of the solid food you eat. The residue, after being thoroughly worked over with acid and other chemicals now enters the small (1½ inches in diameter) intestine which is 30 feet long but it's packaged so neatly you hardly know that it's there.

It's here, in this dark and twisted velvet tunnel, that the final stages of digestion take place. In addition to the enzymes that are normally secreted by the small intestine, there is a liberal injection of bile from the gall bladder, and other enzymes pouring in from the pancreas. Any substance that it's possible to digest will be digested here.

However some substances—for a wide variety of reasons ranging from improper chewing time, to bad combinations of food—simply cannot be digested. Some substances are not meant to be digested—like the fibers of certain vegetables and fruit. They are meant to act as cleansing agents (or bulk gripping agents) for the large intestine.

Anyway, whatever cannot be digested by the small intestine is passed through a special little valve (the ileocecal) into the large (it's larger in diameter) intestine which is only six feet long.

The reason for the special valve is to prevent any rejected matter from coming back into the small intestine. That would be a disaster because the material in the large intestine is very, very poisonous. You would be in big trouble if your personal sewer system started backing up on you.

You see, it's not so much the vegetable matter—it's the undigested protein that's dangerous—particularly meat. This undigested protein that the small intestine shoves out into your large intestine starts to undergo putrefaction almost immediately and it releases a lot of highly toxic material. Now the bacteria in your colon can handle this poisonous substance (for awhile) until it is finally expelled through your rectum.

It's the expulsion that concerns us, mainly. We seem to talk about it—read about it—see it on television—the term being *'regularity'*—and by scaring us half to death they sell us all kinds of perfectly worthless junk called laxatives.

You don't need a laxative to stay 'regular'. You just have to eat decent food and chew it thoroughly and—all things being otherwise normal—you should be as 'regular' as a clock.

When you're not regular—and you find that you are now 'constipated'—fear sets in. Now you're afraid that you will have 'difficulty' in passing a large, hard stool—and you will wind up with 'piles' or 'hemorrhoids'—another favorite subject of the TV huckster.

The simple facts of life is that all you need to get yourself 'cleaned out' is an enema. If you buy one enema bag you can save yourself a lot of money and pain. The money you don't spend on laxatives and the pain you don't get because you don't get piles.

An enema bag, as a little boy I knew used to say, is nothing but a hot water bottle with a long tail. That's about it. The bag holds about two quarts of water—which incidentally is *all* you should ever put in that bag—just water—lukewarm water— *period*. Nothing else—no additives—nothing. Some people recommend everything from soap to salt to god-knows-what. It's asinine to put anything into your body but good old water.

Now the long tail is a rubber tube with a dandy little clamp (which prevents the water coming out unless you want it to) and a nozzle at the end of the tube. You mustn't be afraid of putting this nozzle in your rectum. Most people, the first time they try, tighten up and *naturally* they can't get the nozzle to go in—so they give up in disgust and never use the most useful item in the drugstore—the enema bag.

The main part of the problem is that most people have never even *touched* their rectum (without benefit of a lot of toilet paper between them and their rectum) and that's another asinine left-over of our Puritan heritage. It's *your* rectum, you know—it's not an alien intruder. Get some vaseline jelly and lubricate your rectum liberally. The same with the nozzle. Now insert the nozzle *gently* at the same time you blow gently with your lips forming an "O" and I guarantee the nozzle will slide in.

Now that you know how to use the nozzle, let's get you set up for your enema. The first things you do is rinse out the enema bag with hot water—no soap—just hot water. That's to warm up the bag so that your lukewarm water will stay lukewarm while you're fooling around, getting into position, and so forth.

Your first problem is to find a place to hang the bag—it has to be at least 3 feet higher than you are when you're on your hands and knees with your behind sticking up in the air. Most people forget that the handiest device in your house is a wire coat hanger. Great for hanging things on. If you're lucky enough to have one of those little suction cups with a hook in it—great. Just test it first to make sure that the bag, filled with water, isn't going to be too heavy for it. The filled bag does weigh a bit.

All right. Let's say we've got the bag in position. It's filled with lukewarm water—you're in position—you insert the nozzle as instructed—great.

Know what happens? Nothing. Because you can't find the clamp to unlock and release the water. If you start to laugh at that point—that's not good—because the nozzle shoots out of your rectum like a harpoon.

Second lesson—locate the clamp, try opening and closing it with *one* hand (your other hand will be busy holding the nozzle) and have your hand on the clamp when you get into position.

Third lesson—don't get vaseline on your 'clamp hand' you won't be able to unclamp—you'll start to laugh—and away we go again. If you have vaseline on your hands—wash it off before you start.

Are we ready? All right. Assume the position—I know it's a ridiculous position but it's necessary—besides you're all alone—who's going to see you? Just assume the position, insert the nozzle (gently blowing "O") and unclamp.

When you unclamp, you are going to have a moment of panic. That's normal. Just wait and be patient. It will all feel strange at first and as the water penetrtes deeper you're going to be a wee bit uncomfortable—but that will pass very shortly and you will have a more pleasant feeling.

Eventually, all of the water (2 quarts) will be inside your intestine—just the big one—not the little one—remember the valve? Okay—so you have all the water inside. This is where most people make a big mistake. They get up and sit on the toilet. Wrong. Stay right where you are and massage your stomach gently for a little while. There's no hurry.

And please keep the nozzle in place. That's another mistake people make. They remove it prematurely and—well—you can imagine what *that* does.

Now a word of warning, when you are ready to make your move to the toilet. Do it *slowly* and by the numbers. Remember the nozzle and if you can't seem to have the ability to retain the water, squeeze the cheeks of your behind together (with your clamp hand because your nozzle hand has vaseline on it) and rise *slowly* and carefully. Do not release your cheeks until your body is in position over the toilet. Now sit down and relax and let nature run its course.

A big word of warning at this point. When you have finished evacuating at the toilet, do not assume that you can get dressed. That's wrong. You may *think* you're completely evacuated but you're not. Stick around the bathroom for awhile. Tidy it up, remove the nozzle and wash it carefully. Mop down the walls where the nozzle squirted, do a few knee bends and presto! You will have to leap for the toilet again.

You're going to find that whether you are constipated or not—a good high enema every couple of months is an excellent way to stay regular and healthy.

All right. At this point I think I've belabored your body enough. You should have a fairly good idea of what it's all about; an idea of how not to mistreat it, and an idea of how to unclog your sewer pipes and stay 'regular'.

Now we're going to talk about what to do when you have either loused up your body—or hurt it so badly that somebody else has to fix it up. Remember that most nasty accidents happen in your home. So—one of the first things you have to have in your home is a decent first-aid kit. I don't mean one of those dinky little 5 and 10 monstrosities—I mean a really professional first-aid kit that they sell in either a top drug store or a surgical supply house. Spend a little money on it—because it's one of the best insurance policies you can buy.

The next best insurance policy is to take a first-aid course. They usually have them at the Red Cross Clinics or during the adult-education courses given during summer recess. There are also winter adult education courses that given them.

While you're waiting—drop in at your local book store and pick up a copy of a First-Aid Handbook—or get one from your local library and study it. The knowledge you obtain may help to save the life of a member of your family or a visiting friend, the next time an accident takes place in your home.

The next item on the survival agenda is the emergency ward of your local hospital. Ever been there? Go. At the earliest opportunity. Get in your car and drive there so that you know exaclty how long it takes and exactly how to get there. Go inside. Ask the nurse in charge exactly what the procedure is when you have to bring someone to the emergency ward. Some hospitals have a regular checklist for emergencies. If you have full knowledge of exactly what you must bring—exactly how to get there—the time you save in an emergency can be the difference between life and death.

If you prepare well for an emergency you are in an excellent position to handle one—if it ever arises. When you know exactly what to do, there is little panic—much calm. Panic usually arrives because of helplessness. You won't be helpless. You'll be prepared. Won't you?

The next point is—stop listening and believing the radio and TV commercials which tell you all about the amazing new drugs you can obtain without a prescription. I would be perfectly safe in saying that 99% of the drugs advertised on radio and TV are worthless—and the FDA (Food and Drug Administration) agrees with me. Recent studies by the FDA clearly show that the majority of claims by most commercials for over-the-counter drugs are grossly exaggerated.

It is also a known fact that *combinations* of certain over the counter drugs can cause considerable damage to your system. Which combinations? No one knows until it's too late. Stop trying to medicate yourself. If you eat properly, get enough sleep, fresh air and fresh water—you won't need any kind of drugs—prescribed or over-the-counter.

Just remember that the majority of drugs you can buy *without* a prescription are not designed to *cure* anything. They have only two purposes:

(1) To mask the symptoms—the pain—or the discomfort.
(2) To make billions of dollars for the drug companies.

Let's take them one at a time. Pain or discomfort are important *signals* that something is wrong. Eliminating signals does not eliminate what's wrong with you. Common sense should tell you that. Did you ever *read* the labels on some of the medication you have been taking? The FDA went to a lot of trouble to make sure that the full story is told on those labels. Read them! Read what they say about certain conditions which may make it downright dangerous if you take the medication. Read about dizziness, drowsiness and possible blackouts. Read about facts like high blood pressure, kidney problems, etc. which can be aggravated by these so called 'health aids' (which is the most outrageous title ever devised) and then decide whether you want to introduce this dangerous drug into your system.

I'd like to say something about aspirin. I have always been opposed to the way people take aspirin like candy and I was really happy to hear that the FDA has finally decided that aspirin is not the greatest little pain killer of all time and that it is *not* the safest little pain killer of all time.

The majority of people take aspirin for *headaches*. Right? A headache is a symptom that something is *wrong* with your system. If you have really bad headaches you can bet that there is something really bad going on inside you. Don't keep popping aspirin pills—get a medical checkup and find out what's wrong!

Many headaches are caused by high blood pressure. Bring down your blood pressure and your headaches will disappear.

Some people get headaches because they get tense. Tension can increase your blood pressure and thus—a headache. There are any number of reasons for a headache but there is no valid reason for trying to get 'rid' of one by gobbling aspirin.

People have argued with me about this. I had one woman who became really indignant. *"But the aspirin works,"* she snapped. *"You can't argue with that!"*

"The aspirin works," I told her gently, "because you believe that the aspirin will work—so you relax—and your tension disappears—and so does your headache. But you give the aspirin credit when you should be giving the credit to your sudden relaxation."

"That's nonsense!"

I dropped the subject because there is no sense in trying to reason with a closed mind. The fact is, that many studies have shown that confirmed aspirin users have been given what they *thought* was aspirin (it was just a sugar tablet) and their headaches disappeared. This psycho-somatic effect is well known. There is a whole section of medicine devoted to it.

The lady is wrong. So are you if you take an aspirin as soon as you get a headache. Stop and think for a moment. There are some women who firmly believe that they will get a headache when they ovulate and when they are about to menstruate.

They're absolutely right. They do because they firmly believe that they will and so their computer delivers the headache right on schedule. Several women have argued this concept with me by saying, *"Ah ha! You're wrong because even when I don't know that I'm going to ovulate—the headache comes. So there!"*

Then I remind them that *they* may not know—but their body knows. Just as you might not know what time it is consciously, but your body always knows exactly what time it is. If you want to prove this out, just keep telling yourself, just before you fall asleep that you want to wake up exactly at 5:00 AM. You will.

The next time you get a headache, do the following, before you take your aspirin 'fix': Ask the following questions aloud:

1. Why do I have a headache?
2. Am I tense about something? Is something worrying me?
3. What things could possibly be worrying me right now? (Name all of the possibles. When you come to the right one—if you say it aloud—the headache will vanish on the spot—just like magic.)

If you think that's a lot of nonsense—try it. I convinced a doctor to try it and he called me up in the middle of the night because he was so excited. I told him that now he'd given me a headache and to go back to sleep.

Let's face it—pain, of any kind, is not normal. There has to be a reason for it. Find the reason. It's that simple. Let's suppose you get a terrific back pain. People really get very frightened when they have a back pain. They imagine all sorts of terrible things. That's nonsense. The way we're built and the way we abuse our body, it's amazing we don't have more back pain than we do.

When you get a terrific back pain—usually late in the evening, after you've been sitting—or first thing in the morning when you start to get out of bed—do not panic. Relax and think carefully. Close your eyes and pretend you are in your doctor's office. Do you know what he's going to ask you immediately?

"Have you done anything unusual lately. Lifted anything heavy? Did you slip on something and catch yourself just in time?" and you're going to say,

"Hey—that's right—I was lifting this watermelon and about to put it on top of the refrigerator and my foot slipped and I didn't want to drop the watermelon—How about that?"

And right away you feel a lot better and the doctor tells you take it a little easy—rest and stop picking up those watermelons at your age—and you go away.

You either pay the bill on the way out or the bill arrives in the next month's batch of bills. Save yourself money and save your doctor's time—*think*—the next time you have a back pain. Unless you have a history of back pains, it's a sure bet that you did something unusual and hurt it temporarily.

Any sudden pain, in an unexpected spot, can scare the hell out of you—if you let it. Be calm—do not panic—do not imagine that you have suddenly developed some monstrous disease. Nine times out of ten there is a perfectly logical reason for the pain. A friend of mine rushed to the emergency ward in the middle of the night because he had fallen asleep in his easy chair and woke up with this excruciating pain in his right buttock. I shall not belabor you with the details of what he went through before a cool, young intern made the proper diagnosis. He helped my friend get dressed and told him to go home and check the springs in his easy chair.

The intern explained that the same thing had happened to him after sleeping in a chair that had a broken spring in the seat. That spring had pressed into his buttock and when he awoke the buttock went into a muscle spasm which can be painful and frightening.

So you see? Think before you leap into a panic. There just might be a logical explanation for that pain. The point is—there is a reason. So don't disguise the pain—find out what's causing it. Only after you have eliminated all of the possible non-medical reasons for the pain—should you call your family doctor—or rush to the emergency ward.

FAMILY DOCTOR

Incidentally—do you have a family physician? If you do—you're lucky. But what if you don't? Then get one—soonest. You should have a medical checkup at least once a year. That way there's a record of your internal condition which can be checked against your present condition when something happens. That way there's a comparison of your previous condition and gives doctors a chance to diagnose you.

For example, if you never had an EKG (electrocardiagram) which gives a picture of your heart's particular wave patterns, then it would be difficult (except in extreme cases) to tell whether or not your heart was giving off a normal wave pattern. So the sooner you have a complete checkup (while you're in relatively good health) the sooner your doctor will have something stable to compare your new condition with.

If you haven't a family physician how do you get one? You shop around for one just like you would shop around for a TV repairman or a plumber. You want to find a reliable, personable (you should like your doctor) not too expensive doctor who can keep your health charts up to date. The idea is that you go to a doctor mainly for diagnosis—that means you want an internist who specializes in *diagnostic* medicine rather than in curative medicine—like a surgeon. Your major aim should be prevention rather than rehabilitation. You want to stay out of the hospital by keeping yourself well. Most of the real information your doctor will obtain about you will come from blood analysis. It's amazing how much your blood can tell about your general health—or how much it can tell about the presence of disease.

Most of the time, when you get an examination from your doctor, he's making a shrewd analysis of your general condition from the color of your skin, the tone of your muscles, the sounds of your lungs when you breathe, the whites of your eyes, your fingernail color and things like that. He's also listening to the way you talk, what you say, how you stand and sit. All kinds of general things. The real, deep information, comes from analysis of your blood, urine and feces. They tell the whole story.

Always remember one thing about doctors. While it's true that they have extraordinary training and they are probably extremely well educated—*they are human beings*—not gods. They can make mistakes just like everyone else. They do get tired and forgetful—they do goof occasionally—so take time to tell them everything that you know about yourself.

When your doctor asks you for a medical history—give it to him. Don't just tighten up because he's asking you questions about your previous illnesses. If you have any allergies—tell him about them—it will help him considerably in prescribing certain necessary medication.

Try to pick a doctor you can talk to. Some doctors are so busy they simply haven't got the time to talk to you. Find one who isn't so busy. Try a younger doctor who is just starting up. Don't be afraid that the young doctor hasn't got the depth of experience that the older doctor has. Sometimes the young doctor is more knowledgeable about the latest developments in medicine because the older doctor hasn't got time to keep up with all the latest developments. He may try but there's a limit to the amount of time that a busy doctor can give to seminars and reading about the new advances.

Whether you hire an older doctor or a younger one—ask about his rates. There's no need to be embarrassed about it. You'd ask an auto mechanic his rates, wouldn't you? Okay. Find out in advance exactly what a complete physical checkup will cost you. Shop around and get a lot of rates. Many times you may not have to bother the doctor—just ask the nurse.

Ask around about the doctors you're interested in. Don't take everything you hear as gospel. Take it with a grain of salt. Some people never have a good word for anybody and some people think everybody is wonderful. Get a balance of opinion.

Make an appointment to see the doctor you finally decide upon. Talk to him about *him*. Ask him what his specialty is, if any. Ask for his philosophy of medicine. Don't be afraid, and don't be careless about it. This man may be the man who is ultimately responsible for your entire family's health and well being. Check him out with that thought in mind.

When you decide on the doctor you want, make an appointment to bring the whole family in for a complete medical checkup. It's worth the cost because it will establish medical histories for all of you. It's not intelligent to wait until something goes wrong and then, at a moment, when time counts, to handicap your doctor. Get all of that information about your family's condition into a regular medical history file and then—if something should go wrong, your doctor has a fighting chance to save them.

Regardless of how much you admire and respect your family doctor—always remember that sometimes there is a chance that some medication—for whatever reason—can be wrong for you. If you ever take a prescribed medication and suddenly feel some ill effects from it—stop taking it and immediately contact your doctor and explain what happened. Most doctors will warn you about this possibility—but sometimes you forget the warning or they forget to remind you. You remember—and call him if there are any peculiar side effects.

Now here' a little test for you to take which is designed simply to provoke certain thought. Get a pad and pencil and write down your answers to each of these questions.

MEDICAL VIGILANCE TEST

1. Give the date of your last complete medical checkup.
2. How often do you have headaches? Are they always the same intensity—are some worse than others? What do you do when you have a headache? Do you take aspirin? How much? How often? Do you take tranquilizers? How much? How often?
3. How often do you have back-aches? Are your back-aches always the same intensity? What do you do when you have a back-ache? Do you take over-the-counter pills for the pain? How much? How often?
4. Do you ever become constipated? How often? What do you do to alleviate it? Do you take laxatives? How much and how often? Have you ever taken an enema? If not, now that you know how to take one, will you try it the next time you're constipated?
5. Do you have head-colds? How often? Do you take any medication for a cold? How much and how often? Do they help? Do you follow the regular medical advice for severe colds—rest—stay in bed—drink plenty of liquids, or do you just take medication and keep working? Do you have any idea of *why* you get head-colds?

6. Without looking, can you write down the contents of the medicine chest in your bathroom? When was the last time you checked the contents? Do you keep left over prescription medicine? Why?
7. Is there anything like a first-aid kit in your home or apartment, right now?
8. If an emergency occurred in your home right now, would you know exactly how to obtain an ambulance? Do you know the location of the hospital emergency ward?
9. If a fire broke out in your home or apartment would you know what to do about it?

As I said, these are thought provoking questions. Now is the time to think about the answers. Prevention and preparation are two keys to survival. Forget about the past—you can't do anything about that. It's the future you should be concerned about and you can do something about that—right now.

Incidentally—those left over prescription medicines that you insist on saving are not only useless (they lose effectiveness after a period of time) but they could be dangerous because your physical condition may have changed. Throw them away.

The main thing to remember is that simple, sensible eating, drinking and exercising can keep you young, help you to live longer and—save you a lot of money, at the same time.

Can you imagine the money you would save if you never smoked another cigarette, never bought another batch of aspirin, tranquilizers, over-the-counter cold remedies, and gave up junk food, candy, chewing gum and liquor?

Sit down and add it up. The total amount will make your head spin. The ridiculous part of the whole thing is that all of that garbage is not only costly—it can also wreck your health and shorten your life span considerably.

If you can be honest with yourself and readily admit that up to now you've been deliberately poisoning a perfectly good body, you're half way home. It's not too late to start your rehabilitation proram. Your body—given half a chance—can make an astonishing comeback. If you start now, in less than two weeks you'll not only feel like a new person—you'll look like one too. The difference in your walk, your posture, your skin tone and the sparkle in your eyes will amaze you.

And the improvement in your pocketbook will delight you.

In our next chapter we're going to talk about 'lifestyle' and how it can affect your life expectancy.

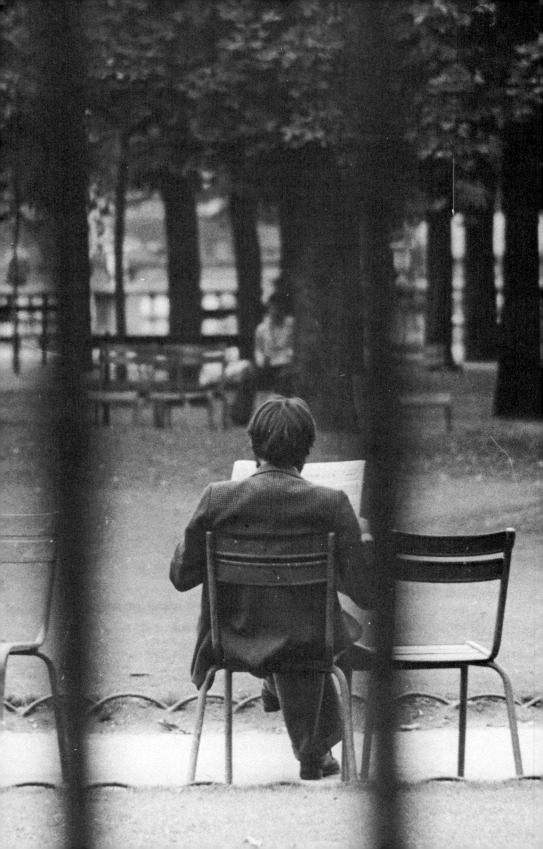

CHAPTER FOUR

LIFESTYLE and
LIFE EXPECTANCY

*Youth is happy because it has the
ability to see beauty. Anyone who
keeps the ability to see beauty
never grows old.*
                    FRANZ KAFKA

The term 'lifestyle' is becoming more and more popular. However, it's just possible that you have never heard the term, or if you have heard about it, never thought much about it.

You should. You have a lifestyle and it just might be that your particular lifestyle is a perfect formula for an early death. Are you interested now? Have I captured your attention? Good. Lifetyle is a very serious business to those who are seriously interested in living rather than just existing, which is what people seem to be doing in this half of the 20th Century.

There is a vast difference between living and existing and it has virtually nothing to do with how much money you have. On the contrary it has to do with your mental attitude towards yourself. That's right—yourself. You are the one who has to make the decision about your lifestyle—no one else can do it for you... *unless you let them do it.*

Let's examine this thing called 'lifestyle' and determine what it is and why it is the way it is. MAYBE IF YOU CAN LOOK AT THE SUBJECT FROM THE OUTSIDE—as an observer—you can begin to understand why it's so important, and what you can do about it in terms of your own life, in the future.

Lifestyle, in essence, is a combination of many different factors which, when added together, present an exact picture of how we live our life. It's a combination of our attitudes, habits, environment (both home and at work), our sex life, our recreation, and our desires for the future.

Let's take lifestyles in general, here in this modern highly technological western world that we live in. What is the opinion of most of our sociologists relative to our lifestyle?

Most of the experts agree that, in the main, our lifestyles are virtually *anti-life.* Or, to put it another way—*suicidal.* Man, it seems, is becoming an endangered species but there is no government agency that can pass laws to protect this particular endangered species.

The irony of our modern society is that the main thrust of our great advances in science have been directed at purely technological problems. It's comparable to a gigantic effort in which we use billions of dollars to create the most perfect legitimate theatre in the world but completely forget to create an area for the audience.

No one can fault the scientific community for their really astonishing technological break-throughs in all branches of scientific effort. They have managed, in a few short years, to accomplish tasks that, less than ten years ago would have been deemed absolutely impossible. At both ends of the scale, the microscopic and the macroscopic, they have extended our ability to see and probe into the secrets of the universe.

Man can now see billions of miles into outer space as easily as he can see across the room; he can also see deep into the structure of matter, almost to the heart of life itself.

And yet, Man himself, is left outside, alone, alienated in a strange world so full of complexities that he will never be able to understand. Is it a wonder that lifestyles are virtually anti-life? Is it surprising that more and more people are becoming (consciously or unconsciously) suicidal?

If you think that's an exaggerated statement let's try a little experiment. We're going to try to construct (with your help) a pattern or a profile, of your particular lifestyle.

You merely have to answer these questions with a TRUE or FALSE. Please think about it before you answer. Give as honest an answer as you can. It's your life we're talking about.

YOUR LIFESTYLE PROFILE

1. The main reason I am living at my present location is because it offers a healthy enjoyable environment.
2. The internal furnishings of my home have been arranged to provide maximum comfort and enjoyment.
3. I have no difficulty in sleeping without medication.
4. The average weather conditions of the area in which I live are highly conducive to my health and well being.
5. Air pollution in the areas in which I work and live are generally said to be within 'safe-limits'.
6. The various areas of my life—such as work, play, meals, sleep and exercise are in harmonious balance.
7. My sex life is healthy and thoroughly enjoyable.
8. I fully enjoy work and look forward to going to work.
9. I enjoy my homelife and look forward to coming home after work.
10. I am rarely bored, depressed, lonely or frustrated.

Score yourself in the following way:

      Give yourself a 5 for every TRUE answer.

      Give yourself a 10 for every FALSE answer.

                          Place total score here _____

Scores of 40 or over indicate that you will have to begin a serious reconstruction of your lifestyle.

If you have finished taking the test you may have some questions in your mind about the validity of the questions asked. Take, for example, the question about *where* you live.

WHERE YOU LIVE

Where you live is highly important to your health. There is a clear link between the quality of the air we breathe and the life we expect to have. For example, in one study that was made in Buffalo, New York a definite relationship was established between air pollution and the increased incidence of cirrhosis of the liver. In addition to being the 7th major cause of death, cirrhosis of the liver can make you feel and look about 30 years older than you actually are.

A study of white American males, living and working in 46 different states showed that those living and working in urban (city) areas had from 1.56 to 2 times the rate of lung cancer as those who worked and lived in rural areas.

Where you live is important to your health. The home or apartment you live in is just as important. A government study conducted in the state of Tennessee clearly showed that 40% of the dwellings tested contained appliances that were giving off dangerous levels of carbon monoxide. That's the same kind of gas given off by your automobile. You know how lethal that can be in a closed garage when the motor is running. Imagine having a high level of carbon monoxide in your home or apartment during the winter time.

Another government survey revealed that as much as 200 pounds of dirty moisture is produced annually in the typical family kitchen. Ever clean off the top of the refrigerator after forgetting to do it for several months? That black gook also goes into your lungs.

Ome of the worst pollutants has only been recognized in recent years as a clear and present danger to your health. That's *noise*. Studies of the effects of noise have shown that noise can cause gastro-intestinal problems, cause a drastic increase in blood pressure (with all the problems *that* entails), have a profound effect upon your moods and emotional outlook and, in general, cause you to age early.

You may not be able to do much about your external noise pollution (other than wear earplugs while traveling through the worst areas of noise) but you can do something about your home environment. The addition of draperies, wall to wall carpets and acoustical, soundproofing wall and ceiling tiles can help to make your home a quieter and more peaceful abode.

Incidentally, if you engage in this kind of soundproofing program, have the minor hazards in your home eliminated at the same time. Have faulty electrical outlets repaired, fix those loose tiles that you keep tripping over, eliminate the long extension cords by having additional electrical outlets installed. Extension cords are a two-way hazard. You can trip over them and you can overload your electrical system by using too many of them (that's a fire hazard).

Make a note to do a periodic safety and hygenic check on your house or apartment. The cleaner your home or apartment is, the less chance for bacteria to breed and feed on you and your family. A cleaner home is not only safer—it's much more pleasant to live in. The exercise will do you almsot as much good as the cleanliness will.

THE AIR YOU BREATHE

Remember that fresh air is a *must* the year round. Stale air, like stale water, is bad for your system and can lead to racking headaches if continued over a period of time. Air your house or apartment periodically and make certain that there is always a supply of clean fresh air.

We mentioned 'climate and weather conditions' in our Lifestyle Profile. Just how important are they to good health? Oddly enough, most climates and weather conditions could be easily adjusted to—*if we lived outdoors*. Our body has all the equipment necessary to adjust to virtually every kind of weather condition ranging from extremely cold to the extremely hot. However, we do not live outdoors, we live indoors in what has been described as a 'controlled environment' which implies that it's 'good for you.' Unfortunately it is not good for you at all. A human being is a balanced organism that has been conditioned over a million years to react to natural conditions with ease. We are at our best when we are in tune with nature; at our worst in an artificial environment.

Just consider the 'cabin fever' that develops during a long, hard, bitter winter, when we tend to stay indoors for long period of time. Man requires fresh air and sunlight (even sunlight that's filtered through clouds) because eventually he will sicken and die as an indoor houseplant. When you consider that the law provides that all criminals in prisons and various penitentiaries must be allowed to walk and exercise outdoors at least once a day, then you can appreciate the necessity of giving yourself the same opportunity.

ENVIRONMENT

Of late, there is a greater emphasis on artificial environment, both in the home and at work, and people are finding that, with the exception of summer vacations, they spend less and less time in natural surroundings with fresh air and sunlight.

You pay a high price for 'creature comfort' offered by air conditioning and central heating. Not just in terms of physical debilitation but in your mental health as well. That's because you are not in harmony with nature, as you were meant to live. Your body suffers in various ways ranging from a drastic change in your basal metabolism—which is the standard energy turnover of your body at a low level of activity . . . to the natural rhythm of your various glands and organs.

There are several marked effects of continuous living and working in artificial environments. One of the most noticeable effects is the difference in skin tone. There is a pallor, an absence of life in the skin and in the eyes of a person who has become an indoor person.

Motor activity is also markedly different. The indoor person tends to be sluggish, slow moving and perpetually tired (very similar to people with sluggish livers).

The appetite usually is low or absent and food tends to be tasteless. In general, there is a lowering of vitality and most certainly there is a severe change in mental outlook.

BOREDOM AND DEATH

That brings us to the most dangerous of attitudes and that is *boredom*. It is entirely possible to be *bored to death*. I mean that quite literally. Man is, from birth to death, perched quite precariously on a thin line that separates his wish to live from his wish to die. Boredom is a danger sign. It means that the death wish is growing stronger and the wish to live is growing weaker. The tendency towards death influences the body to comply with the death wish. A chain of events will begin to take place and the person will begin to become less and less active and the desire to live begins to wane. Inactivity is a key to early aging and early death.

Remember that boredom is a choice. A person choose to be bored, rather than discovers that boredom has simply happened. If you have become bored with your job, with your home, with your family, then realize that this is your choice and that it can be changed with very little effort. However, you have to make the effort, no one can do it for you.

Think very carefully. Are you bored with your job? With your life in general? With your mate and/or your children?

Are you indifferent to food? Are your forced to drag yourself from bed each morning with a groan and hate the idea of going to work? When the end of the work day comes are you hating the idea of going home? Then you'd better realize something in a great big hurry before it's too late.

You are choosing to die, rather than live.

HOW TO CHANGE

If you want to change that, fast, and with little effort, take a long walk on your lunch hour. Don't smoke during the walk. Just breathe in the air and enjoy the sunshine. Don't try to think about anything, just enjoy being alive for a change.

When your work day is over, or perhaps a half hour before, call your wife or husband and suggest that you go out for dinner. It needn't be an expensive restaurant, just a decent one with decent food that you can both enjoy.

You'll be amazed at what a difference those two 'changes' will make in your outlook. Here are a few more suggestions that can help immensely. Set your alarm clock an hour ahead and get up an hour earlier than usual. Get washed, dressed, drink a glass of orange juice or grapefruit juice and then take a short walk. Even a city can be quite beautiful and quiet early in the morning. If you life in the country it's astonishing how lovely everything is early in the morning.

You'll find, after that short walk, that you have a keen, new appetite and can really put away a nourishing breakfast. Leave for work a little early and look at everything on the way to work as though you have never seen it all before. You might be surprised to find that you really haven't looked at everything.

Now, because you're early and have plenty of time, you'll be more relaxed and able to enjoy simple sights almost with a child-like delight. Life can be beautiful if you give it a chance.

The trick of living is to become involved with life, to learn to embrace life like a brand new lover who is full of unexpected delights. It really doesn't require money to be completely happy with life. In fact, money sometimes gets in the way *because people with money believe that they can buy pleasure* when the truth is that pleasure, real pleasure is offered free by life itself to anyone with the wit to find it.

Let's just take the magnificence of an early morning in Spring with a fantastic sunrise on the horizon. This is one of nature's most astonishing presents. It makes anything that Man is capable of, seem puny and ineffectual. It really is one of the greatest shows on Earth—and it's free. No millionaire owns the gorgeous sunrise—it's a gift to every human being.

How many sunrises have you ever seen? Or have you been too engrossed in looking down? Or so caught up with your internal unhappiness that you've been walking around with your eyes closed. So closed up that you have never touched the petal of a flower or inhaled the delicate fragrance and marvelled that nature can, with ease, create beauty of sight and aroma that Man can only feebly imitate.

Open yourself up to life and the riches of living that cost nothing but are priceless beyond the wealth of any man. All of life is waiting for you to take freely without limit other than the limits you set upon yourself.

If you really want to overcome boredom *(and you have to want to)* then the simplest way is to design a program of activity for yourself. Activity is the first enemy of boredom.

The way to design that program is set up a Pleasure Ledger which simply means to make a list of all the things that you would really like to do. Please do not limit yourself with the thought that you cannot possibly afford to do most of these things. Pretend that there is no question of money involved.

I'll give you an idea of what a Pleasure Ledger should look like and then you can make your own list up. Think of it as a sort of wishing game like the "If I had a million" kind of game, where you could wish for just about anything under the sun. Perhaps you could pretend that you found a bottle with a genie in it—or Aladdin's magic lamp. Just let your imagination run riot and you've got the idea.

PLEASURE LEDGER

1. Deep sea diving fascinates me. I'd like to be able to take a few voyages with Jacques Costeau and his crew and actually experience some of their adventures.
2. Space travel must be an awesome experience. I'd like to pilot a space craft and take a trip like the one shown in Stanley Kubric's film "2001."
3. I've always admired people who are able to paint portraits and landscapes. I'd like to study painting and be able to create real masterpieces in oil or tempera.

Are you beginning to get the idea? Now I'll admit that these are fairly mundane desires, but they're real desires and that's what's important. You should put down things that really turn you on—regardless of what they are. Treat your pleasure ledger like a very personal diary. No one but you will ever see it, so you can really let yourself go. Fantasize if you want to. Do you have hidden sexual desires—let them all hang out. Just loosen up and write down all the things that you would like to do, regardless of how strange or peculiar they might seem to you. Get them all down on paper and you will discover that many of them are quite attainable. *Mainly let this be a fun project that you can really enjoy.*

You'll be amazed at the pleasure it will give you once you start to do it. All it takes is a pencil, some paper and your own fertile imagination.

LONELINESS

Loneliness is, without a doubt, one of the worst afflictions that can befall a human being. Unless you have actually had the experience yourself, you cannot possibly imagine the depth of despair that loneliness can produce. Even those people who work to alleviate the suffering of lonely people cannot fully realize what a bottomless pit of agony this state induces.

Here and there, in a painting or a photograph, you might catch just a glimpse, a hint, and if you are very perceptive, a chill of fear ripples through you, and then you shudder slightly at the thought of what it must be like. Then, ever so quickly, you shake off the feeling and think of more pleasant things.

What we see (or think we see) at that moment, is just the tiny tip of an enormous iceberg, which spreads below the surface of our understanding and encompasses millions of people. To understand why this is such a widespread affliction, you have to look at loneliness as a condition with many dimensions, many faces, many causes. It is not a simple affliction.

Let's start with the most familiar form of loneliness—the kind that's caused by 'solitary confinement'. That seems like a fairly simple term. It is not simple. I have seen hardened criminals turn pale and shake with terror at the mere threat of solitary confinement. They know the meaning behind those words. So do the untold hundreds of thousands of innocent, helpless, infirm, elderly people who are forced to live in a cheerless box of a room in solitary confinement. Many of them have only the brief visit of a health agency nurse or volunteer to look forward to. But what about all the other lonely hours?

Those helpless people are the involuntary victims of their 'solitary confinement'. There are also voluntary inhabitants of that lonely hell. Men and women who could leave but won't.

They *choose* to be lonely but don't realize that they have made a choice. They think they're a victim of circumstance. They're not and yet they suffer just as much as the people who have no other choice. Many of these lonely people live in the most populated cities on this Earth. It would seem impossible for them to be lonely and yet they are. They have stepped out of the mainstream of life. They have become spectators instead of participants. They are no longer involved with life.

I have met several hundred 'lonely by choice' people over the years and they have all, almost without exception, said,

"How lucky you are! How wonderful it must be to have so many friends, so many interests!"

I tell them all the same thing that I'm going to tell you.

"Luck has nothing to do with it. It's choice. I choose to embrace life. I choose to meet people, to become involved with people, to become involved with life. You can too."

"How?" they cry. *"How? I don't know how!"*

"It's very simple," I say. "Just *volunteer*."

That's right—volunteer to help someone who can't help himself. Give your time to make someone else's live brighter. The need for volunteers in our society is overwhelming. The Red Cross, March of Dimes, Muscular Dystrophy, Cystic Fibrosis, all of the national health agencies are crying out for volunteers. Most of the hospitals in this nation could not continue to operate if it were not for volunteers—and they need all they can get.

Visit one of these agencies, offer to give a few hours of your time. They will embrace you with both arms. You will find yourself needed. You will, in a short time, meet and make friends with more people of both sexes than you could possibly meet in ten lifetimes of ordinary social life. You will never be lonely or bored again and, more importantly, you will have contributed to someone else's happiness at the same time.

TIME TO READ

One of the things that always surprises me is the statement *"I'd love to be able to read books, but I just can't seem to find the time to do it."*

Whenever I hear that, my first response is—*make* the time. Get up an hour early, while everyone is sleeping, and read for an hour. If you do that regularly, you can read every book you've ever wanted to read and you'll find that you've become a really interesting person in the process.

Another trick is to take a book in the bathroom with you. Don't just sit there—read! You'll find that it's a lot healthier too because you won't have a tendency to rush your bowel movements which is an unhealthy thing to do. So do take a book with you to the bathroom. That way you'll satisfy both the body and the mind at the same time.

Take a book to work with you and read during your lunch period. You'll find yourself eating more slowly and enjoying your food more and you'll be feeding your mind at the same time, which isn't a bad idea at all.

Get up early on Sunday mornings and take a book to the park or the waterfront or someplace quiet and spend an hour or two reading and enjoying the fresh air.

Just remember, if you really want to read, you can always arrange an hour or two somewhere by making a slight adjustment in your lifestyle. Books are free, you know. The library is just delighted to have you borrow them. That's what they're there for.

NEW LEARNING

Another thing that's really great fun is to learn something. Just pick a subject. It doesn't matter what. Say it's computers, for example. You'd like to know a lot more about them. Just visit your public library and look up 'computers' in the index file. You'll probably find a half dozen books ranging in complexity from simple language to highly esoteric. Take out the book that suits your language style and read it. You'll be amazed at how much you can learn all by yourself.

There are books on just about every kind of activity. Books that can teach you how to do it—or just how to understand it. Take ceramics, for example. It's one of the easiest, simplest and least expensive hobbies you can get into. In almost every community, there is a ceramics store which offers free lessons because they want you to buy their supplies (which are really quite inexpensive). You really haven't lived until you have actually created your own mug, decorated it, fired it in the store's kiln and then later on, made a drink in it and used it. There's an almost atavistic pleasure in using something that you have created.

Let's suppose that you have a longing to be part of a theatre group—not necessarily as an actor—possibly as a scenic designer or a costume designer—a lighting director—anything. Here again there is hardly a community that doesn't have a little theatre group. They are delighted to receive volunteers in any capacity.

If there isn't a theatre group in your community—study up on the subject of how you start one—and start one.

As I said before, there is a lot of sheer pleasure in simply living to do the things you really want to do. All you have to do to find out what you want to do is ask yourself. Write down all your desires in that pleasure ledger and then start doing them. I'm willing to bet that in no time at all you're going to realize that if you had a thousand years to live you couldn't possibly do all the things you want to do.

You're just going to be too busy to be bothered with boredom, because you're going to be enjoying life too much. Which is the way it's supposed to be. Life is for living—not brooding. Life is for giving and receiving pleasure.

Start enjoying. Because in our next chapter we're going to show you how to eat so that you can enjoy a longer life.

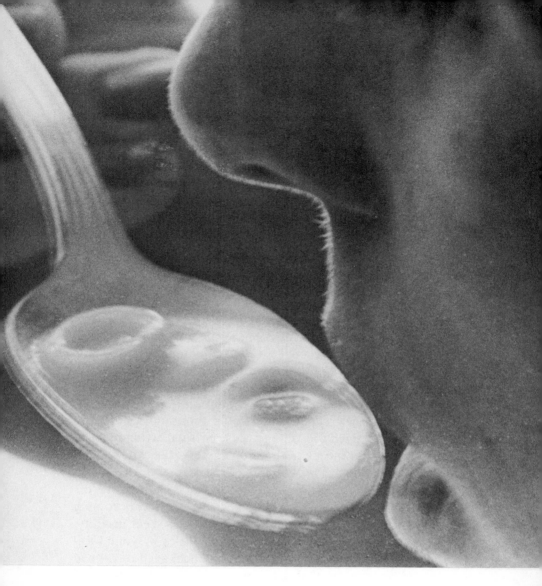

CHAPTER FIVE

WHAT YOU EAT
IS HOW YOU AGE

*The stresses of modern life have
made the need for adequate nutrition
greater than ever.*
ADELL DAVIS

THE SUPERMARKET AGE

In this chapter we're going to deal with one of the most important factors that govern good health and long life—that's *food*. At the same time we are probably going to raise considerable controversy because there is a great deal wrong with the way we, in America, are eating. Most of the fault lies not in ourselves but in our food providers. Let's see why.

When historians write about this period in American history they will undoubtedly dub it 'The Age of the Supermarket' and they will be close to hitting the mark. I think my personal preference would be the 'Age of the Great Food Ripoff' because, to paraphrase good old Winston Churchill,

"Never has so much been offered that provided so little."

When you travel the length and breadth of America as I have, year after year, you become aware of one fact of life. There is, in virtually every decent sized community, at least one supermarket. It will be either a national chain supermarket or a variation of the IGA (Independent Grocers Association) supermarket. Sometimes in some communities there are both.

Either way, these supermarkets offer thousands of brightly packaged, processed foods. I use the term 'food' with tongue in cheek because, in the main, they don't deserve the title. I would prefer to call them **PPOP** items (Processed, Packaged and Overpriced) that pass as food that have contributed to the sorry spectacle of the richest nation on earth rapidly becoming the most undernourished nation on earth. It's sheer insanity.

Just walk down the brightly lighted aisles in your local supermarket and pick up just about any packaged or canned item and read the label aloud (if you can pronounce the multi syllabic chemicals) and listen to what you are reading:

This product contains sodium caseinate, mono and diglycerides, dipostassium phosphate, sodium silicate aluminate, BHT and BHA and on and on—and almost nothing about the *food* it is supposed to contain.

One of the worst offenders is the cereal manufacturers. Some wit once remarked that there was more nutrition and wholesome flavor and goodness in the *box* than there was in the cereal itself. He recommended tearing up the box and sprinkling it with sugar and milk and eating *that* instead of the garbage that posed as cereal. He was right as rain.

If just a quarter of the money spent on outrageous advertising claims and fancy multi-colored packaging, was spent on creating a nutritious cereal, we'd all be better off. However, that's not the way things are done.

We simply cannot expect that the giant corporations that are engaged in the 'food processing' business are going to be concerned with our health and well being. They're in business to make money—not to help us live longer. We have to do that.

DEFENSIVE BUYING

You've heard the expression that 'defensive driving' is the best way to stay alive on the highways? Well, we're going to do a little teaching about 'defensive buying' when you visit your good old neighborhood supermarket.

Just as you wouldn't pick up a strange medicine and swallow it, don't pick up chemicalized food and swallow it unless you enjoy playing 'russian roulette' because that's exactly what you're doing. If you don't know what the chemicals are (that are listed on the label) don't swallow them—it's that simple. There are a number of products on the market now that state in large clear print—nothing artificial—no chemicals added.

Know why? Because people are beginning to refuse to eat the chemicalized garbage that's being offered. Eventually, when enough people refuse, the giant corporations will change their ways. Obviously not enough people have, as yet, which is why all that junk is still being sold. But, until the change comes— you start to buy your food 'defensively' and live longer.

TO STAY YOUNG

Now suppose that I told you that there was a substance that could give you virtually unlimited energy (regardless of your age) and that there was a companion substance that could make you look younger—stay younger and live longer?

You probably wouldn't believe me—or if you did, you'd probably expect to pay a fortune for these two substances. Well, you can believe me because they both exist—and you don't have to pay a fortune to get them.

The two substances are DNA and RNA—they're tongue twisters but here they are—deoxyribonucleic acid (DNA) and ribonucleic acid (RNA) and they're part of the most important discoveries man has made with reference to health, energy, youth and long life. Here's why:

Any food that's rich in nucleic acid is a vital source of energy for our body's cells. Now the building blocks of the nucleic acids are called nucleotides. Any food with these substances seem to contribute to youthful looking skin and help a person to stay younger looking longer.

The key to repairing damaged cells in your body is a substance called adenosine triphosphate (ATP). Nucleic acids increase the production of ATP in your body.

All right? Then here are the foods that you should add to your diet if you want the benefits of DNA and RNA:

CALVES LIVER, SARDINES, SALMON, SHRIMP, LOBSTER, CLAMS and OYSTERS, BEEF KIDNEYS, PINTO and LIMA BEANS, LENTIL, POULTRY, SPINACH, MUSH-ROOMS, OATMEAL, ONIONS, ASPARAGUS, NUTS, WHEAT GERM, RADISHES, LAMB'S LIVER and HEART, BEETS (which contain amino acids which help the body to create more nucleic acid of its own).

Sardines, incidentally, happen to be one of the best forms of protein for dieters who want to lose weight and stay healthy at the same time. Ask your dietician to give you a rundown on sardines, the complete story will fascinate you. And they are really low priced, too!

Now let's get down to basics about food. There are only four basic categories and they are:
1. Meat and fish
2. Vegetables and fruit
3. Milk and dairy products
4. Breads and cereals

The key word in proper nutrition is *balance*. Just remember balance and moderation and you have it made. If you decide that you want to start feeling healthy and filled with energy then you have to start planning to eat properly. That means you have to start eating *real food* and eliminate the over-refined chemically filled, junk food that fills the shelves of your local supermarket. You will have to give up refined sugar that offers false, limited energy and makes you fat. A number of new theories now advance the idea that sugar, rather than fats are a major cause of heart disease. All I know is that refined sugar is bad for you. You can get all the sugar you want or need from natural sources like fruit and fruit juices.

In yoga, the two opposing forces of life are yang and yin. If we speak of food (and balance) consider 'yin' as acidity—and yang as alkalinity. If you can balance your food so that you have a combination of both acid and alkaline, then you're beginning to learn the secret of a healthy long life.

You must select your food as fuel for your body. Just as you wouldn't think of using a low octane gasoline in your car which is designed for high octane gas (because you'd damage the engine)—think about the damage you can cause to your body's priceless engine with the addition of improper fuel (food).

Do you know exactly what your eating habits are? Do you have any idea whether your meals are properly balanced? Here's a little TRUE or FALSE quiz that you can take, which may give you some surprises. Just put an honest T or F next to each question.

EATING HABIT QUIZ

1. I always have sugar in my coffee or tea.
2. I always sprinkle sugar on my cereal in the morning.
3. I usually skip breakfast because I have no appetite.
4. At lunchtime I usually have a sandwich or a hamburger.
5. I like sandwiches and have bread and butter at meals.
6. I keep pretzels, potato chips, cookies and cake around for a snack between meals or while I'm watching TV.
7. I generally drink a couple of beers while watching TV because beer is really a food, you know?
8. I like fried foods like fried eggs or french fries.
9. When I want to lose weight or cut down I just skip breakfast and lunch and have just one meal at night.
10. I drink about 5 or 6 cups of coffee (or tea) a day.

Give yourself 10 for each TRUE answer
Give yourself 5 for each FALSE answer

TOTAL _____

Remember that any TRUE answer
should be regarded as detrimental to health and long life.

Now I'm not going to lecture you about your bad habits. You know they're bad without my telling you. You know that coffee and tea, even in moderation, are not good for you. Refined sugar is poison to your system. Natural honey would be a much better substitute on your cereal. If you eat a lot of bread and sandwiches you're choking your liver to death. Fried fats are extremely tough on your system.

All right. I'll stop and instead I'll tell you about some of the life-giving foods—the 17 Live Foods that you should always include in your diet. If you do—you'll be amazed at how healthy and young looking you'll become in a very short while.

LIVE FOODS

1. Wheat germ
2. Yogurt
3. Fresh fruit
4. Fresh fish
5. Seeds and nuts
6. Raw vegetables
7. Vinegar
8. Raw Eggs
9. Live oysters
10. Live clams
11. Cheese (natural not processed)
12. Soybeans
13. Fresh bean sprouts
14. Honey
15. Garlic
16. Fresh milk
17. Yeast (important powerhouse of all B vitamins)

Naturally, these are not the only foods you need in your diet, but they should be *included* in your diet not only because they are exceptionally good for you, but because they are delicious.

I should also have included water (fresh water) on that list. You should have at least two or three glasses of fresh water every day. It's vitally necessary to permit your body to carry on the many chemical transformations during the day.

FASTING

There has been a lot of controversy about fasting. While most doctors are opposed to it, quite recently a number of doctors have expressed the opinion that fasting isn't a bad idea. They don't feel that it can do any harm.

I can agree with that only in part. I know that many of you will write and tell me that the American Indian was a great believer in fasting, and look what great shape he was in.

You're absolutely right, but you have to realize that the American Indian *was in great shape to begin with*. His fasting was more ceremonial and spiritual than part of a reducing diet. He didn't need to stay in shape. He was in great shape.

If you are, and your doctor says it's all right—then fast if that's what you want to do. I can only express my opinion to those people who are not in good shape—don't do it.

Remember what happens when you fast. First of all you deny the vital protein that your body needs for repairs. You also deny your body the B complex vitamins your body needs every day of your life as well as the Vitamin C it cannot manufacture.

If you fast, for any length of time, you'd better have help close at hand because you can faint quite easily after a period of time without food. You should never attempt to fast for extremely long periods of time because you can die, quite suddenly from lack of protein.

In any event, certainly check with your doctor before attempting any fasting or 'crash' diets because they can be extremely dangerous unless you know what you're doing.

HEALTH RECIPES

It was not my intention to turn this book into a cookbook or a diet book. The concept is a book that will help you to reshape your life through proper eating habits, proper attitudes and new insight. All together, this book should help you to lead a healthier, happier and longer life.

However, there is no reason why I can't give you a couple of simple recipes for some delicious, nutritious and very inexpensive treats that you can make and enjoy at home any time you're in the mood.

I don't know whether you've ever picked up a recipe and just made something for the fun of it—but it is fun, particularly when you eat what you've made. It's even more fun when you make something that you usually have to pay money for— some times a lot more money than you should pay.

The best part of making something is that you know exactly what kind of ingredients went into it—the exact condition of the kitchen it was made in (something we are rather shocked to learn about when we hear investigations into manufacturers kitchens) and—as I said—these foods generally cost you less.

The first recipe I'm going to give you is for **yogurt**. You may have never tasted yogurt before—if so you're in for a big surprise. It's really delicious. It's also one of the oldest foods around. We are told that Moses served it to his guests and that Ghengis Khan fed it to his fabulous armies that overran the entire world at one time. So it has a long, long history.

In addition to being almost indecently delicious, yogurt is extremely low in calories and very high in protein. It's a superb food that does wonders for your highly important digestive system and once you try it, you'll be hooked for life.

HOW TO MAKE BULGARIAN YOGURT

For 1 quart of yogurt, you will need
1 quart of milk
3 heaping tablespoons yogurt (commercial)

Heat saucepan of milk until *almost* boiling, then pour into crockery bowl. When the milk has cooled to slightly warmer than lukewarm (hot, but not enough to burn) add yogurt culture (which has been brought to room temperature). Stir gently. Cover and wrap bowl in a blanket or large towel for at least six hours (preferably overnight). Refrigerate to store.

Be sure to reserve ½ cup of your fresh new yogurt to be used as culture for your next homemade batch. Once you start, you need never buy commercial yogurt again!

Enjoy it plain, or add a spoonful of fruit, honey or berries for healthful variety and delicious eating.

Serve an avocado, a baked potato, hot green peas or a bed of lettuce topped with a spoon of creamy white yogurt.

Create a piquant yogurt sauce with a pinch of garlic, dill, parsley, basil or other herbs.

Yogurt is often dubbed "one of the five wonder foods". Make it a part of your menu planning.

Whole grain are an important part of healthful eating.

RICE is the staple food of over half the human race and its importance cannot be overestimated. Seek brown rice for full food value, or enjoy wild rice or yellow grain patna rice (the latter is particularly good for cereals and puddings). Be creative when cooking with grains . . . don't forget what we said about the importance of flavor and appeal. For example:

RICE AND RAISIN MOUSSE

⅓ cup brown rice
3½ cups milk
1 tablespoon gelatin
¼ cup light brown sugar

3 tablespoons cold water
1 teaspoon vanilla
1 teaspoon almond extract
1 cup whipped cream
1 cup raisins

After washing rice, cook covered in double boiler until tender, stirring occasionally. (Approximately 1 hour). Add sugar and gelatin which has soaked 3 minutes in cold water. Fold in raisins, flavorings and whipped cream. Spoon into fancy dish or mold and chill.

Whole grain cookery *can* be *elegant* as well as healthful!

WHOLE GRAIN WHEAT makes a hearty porridge for a cold winter morning and a healthy vigorous day.

WHOLE-GRAIN WHEAT PORRIDGE

2 cups whole grain wheat
2 teaspoons salt
4 cups water

Soak grain for 12 hours. Drain. Add 4 cups water and bring to a boil. Add salt and simmer over a very low flame for 12 hours, stirring occasionally. Serve with honey and cream.

CORN is valued today as it was among the American Indians when our country was new. Try these corn pancakes for nutritious eating and really unique flavor.

NATURE'S CORN PANCAKES

1 cup corn meal
½ teaspoon salt
1 egg beaten

½ teaspoon soda
1 teaspoon melted butter
¼ cup sour cream

Sift all the dry ingredients and combine with all the liquid ingredients (after the liquids have been beaten together). Fry on a hot greased griddle. Makes 8 cakes.

(Try a spoon of your fresh yogurt on these!)

If you have a thing about bread, then bake your own and enjoy a really nutritious and delicious bread that's good for you! Here's a simple recipe that will make a really great bread.

HARVEST PUMPKIN BREAD

½	cup of warm water	½	cup dried skim milk
1	teaspoon brown sugar	½	cup soft butter
¼	teaspoon ginger	1½	teaspoons salt
2	packages dry yeast	1	teaspoon cinnamon
¾	cup warm water	1	cup cooked sieved pumpkin
½	cup brown sugar	4	cups whole grain flour
1	cup of flour		

Combine the first four ingredients and let stand in a warm place until bubbling nicely. In a large bowl stir together ¾ cup warm water, ½ cup brown sugar, 1 cup flour, and ½ cup dried skim milk. Add the yeast mixture and beat well. Add ½ cup soft butter, 1½ teaspoons salt, 1 teaspoon cinnamon, 1 cup pumpkin and 3 cups whole grain flour. Stir until the dough clears the bowl. Spread the remaining 1 cup of whole grain flour on pastry board, turn out dough and knead thoroughly, using a little more flour, if necessary, to make a smooth, non-sticky dough.

Return to bowl, grease top of dough with butter, cover and let stand in a warm place until double in bulk. Turn out of bowl, knead lightly, divide in half and form loaves of any desired shape.

Brush tops of loaves lightly with melted butter. Let rise until double in bulk. Bake in oven preheated to 350°F for about 45 minutes.

About 10 minutes before the end of the baking period, brush tops of loaves with evaporated milk so that they will brown to a lovely russet shade.

NOTE: The length of time necessary to allow dough to double in bulk depends upon temperature, amount of yeast, richness of dough and king of flour used.

Vegetables can be exciting as well as nutritious. No gourmet could ask for more than...

GLAZED CARROTS WITH ONIONS AND WHITE GRAPES

1   bunch (medium) carrots
1   cup cooked (boiled) onions
1   cup seedless grapes, halved
4   tablespoons white corn syrup
1   tablespoon lemon juice
1½ tablespoons brown sugar
¼   teaspoon salt
1   tablespoon chopped parsley

1. Cut carrots into strips. Cook and drain.
2. Combine carrots and onions in shallow baking dish, with the cup of grapes.
3. Make mix of syrup, brown sugar, salt and lemon juice. Bring to a boil in small saucepan.
4. Pour syrup over vegetables and bake in 400°F oven for 10-15 minutes, turning once.
5. Serve garnished with a circle of parsley.

If you want a delicious and nutritious dessert, try:

SOY PUMPKIN PUDDING

6 tablespoons honey
½ cup whole wheat pastry flour
¼ teaspoon salt
1¼ cup cooked pumpkin
1 teaspoon vanilla
1½ cups soy milk

Blend all ingredients together and bake in preheated 350°F oven for 45 minutes. Individual molds may be used. Pudding is delicious topped with any fruit sauce.

BAKED GRAPEFRUIT

2 Grapefruits—halved
2 tablespoons honey
1 lemon

Drizzle honey over grapefruit halves, squeeze small amount of lemon juice over each half, bake under broiler for 5 minutes.

VEGETABLE TART

2	tablespoons chopped onion	2	tablespoons butter
1	tablespoon flour	1½	teaspoons salt
⅛	teaspoon pepper	1	egg slightly beaten
1	cup cooked peas	½	cup cooked corn
	& carrots	¼	cup cooked lima beans
½	cup cooked green beans	1	cup mashed potatoes
¾	cup vegetable cooking water	2	tablespoons grated Parmesan cheese

Saute onion in butter until golden. Add flour, salt and pepper, blending well. Add vegetables with ¾ cup of vegetable cooking liquid and simmer until the mixture thickens, stirring constantly. Pour into greased casserole. Beat egg and potato until light. Spread over vegetable mixture, using pastry tube if desired. Sprinkle with cheese and paprika. Bake in preheated 375°F oven until brown.

If you enjoy doing these kinds of recipes then by all means visit your nearest health food store where you can get books filled with natural cooking recipes.

Meanwhile I would like to discuss vitamins with you. I certainly couldn't close this chapter on food without talking about them. There are only three ways to get vitamins.

1. From the *natural foods* in which they are found.
2. From *natural extracts* from natural foods.
3. From *man-made synthetic* vitamins.

Naturally, the best place to get your vitamins is directly from the foods that contain them. So I am going to give you a guided tour of vitamins and where they are found. If you get your vitamins this way you will not only be healthier but you'll save an awful lot of money.

Remember—the list that I'm going to give you is just about the last word on vitamins as far as your natural sources go. If you get your vitamins naturally you'll never have to worry about whether you are eating properly again—you will be.

YOUR VITAMIN GUIDE

Vitamin	What it's for	Where you find it
A	It's important for good eyesight and night vision Gives you a decent skin and protects tissues in your nose, mouth, throat and lungs. Helps prevent infection. Helps in the growth and repair of tissue. Stores in liver so it's not necessary to take any supplements unless you know you're deficient.	All dark green vegetables. All yellow vegetables like yams, sweet potatoes, and carrots. Incidentally you have to juice, chop, grate or cook carrots to release vitamin A—so stop eating them raw unless you chew them really thoroughly. Cooking won't hurt the vitamin but air and sunlight will. So store them in the refrigerator. If you have them in salads don't use too much salad dressing or you'll make vitamin absorption difficult.
B Complex	Converts carbohydrates into glucose which the body burns to produce energy. Important for muscle tone, and for the liver, eyes, skin, mouth and hair.	Whole grains, green leafy vegetables, brewers yeast all meat organs. Since B complex is really 13 separate vitamins and you must have all of them and you need B complex every day, it's best to get it from natural sources.
B1	Also known as Thiamine this vitamin is vital to your nervous system, heart and liver. Also needed to convert starch and sugar into glucose.	Brown rice (not white) in wheat germ, in whole wheat bread (not white bread) in brewers yeast, sunflower seeds raw peanuts (not roasted) in whole grains and beans.
B2	Also called Riboflavin. Helps vision, gives you clear, healthy eyes. Works with enzymes to assist cells in oxygen usage. Helps to break down fats, carbohydrates and protein.	Liver, whole milk, milk products, buttermilk and yogurt, brewers yeast, wheat germ, almonds, wild rice, mushrooms and turnip greens.
B6	Pyridoxine. Helps form anti-bodies and red blood cells. Important to use of energy in the brain and central nervous system.	Whole grains, wheat germ nuts and brewers yeast.
B12	Cobalamine. Needed for the formation of red cells. Its essential for normal function of all body cells especially in bone marrow, gastrointestinal tract and nervous tissue.	Meat, fish, milk and milk products, eggs, soybeans

89

Vitamin	What it's for	Where you find it
Biotin	Helps the body use amino acids folic acid, pantothenic acid and B12. Helps burn up fatty acids and carbohydrates for body heat, and energy.	Organ meats, brewers yeast and whole grains
Choline	It's the main ingredient of lecithin which helps move fats from liver to cells. Plays a part in transmitting nerve impulses.	Eggs, wheat germ, fish, peanuts, beans, peas and organ meats.
Folic Acid	Folacin. Aids in formation of nucleic acid and red blood cells. Helps in forming heme which is the iron-containing protein in hemoglobin.	Brewers yeast, gland meat, green, leafy vegetables
Inositol	Works with Choline to help form Lecithin which moves fats from the liver to cells.	Whole grains, vegetables, nuts, citrus fruits and organ meats
Niacin	Helps break down and use of proteins, fats, carbohydrates. Helps maintain physical and mental health. Maintains the health of the skin, tongue and digestive system.	Peanuts, organ meats, Turkey and chicken. Milk and milk products, Meat and fish, Whole grains
PABA	Para-Aminobenzoic Acid. Helps intestinal bacteria produce folic acid which helps produce pantothenic acid. Helps breakdown and use of proteins. Helps to form red blood cells.	Organ meats and green leafy vegetables.
Panto-thenic Acid	Helps the functioning of the adrenal gland which affects growth. Also helps maintain healthy skin and nerves. Helps to release energy from protein, fats and carbohydrates. Participates with other vitamins to withstand stress.	Brewers yeasts, organ meats, eggs and grains.
B15	Pangamic Acid. Said to be effective in the treatment of hypoxia (insufficient supply of oxygen to cells).	Brewers yeast and seeds.

Vitamin	What it's for	Where you find it
C	Ascorbic Acid. Maintains collagen, a protein needed for the formation of skin ligaments and bones. Heals wounds, forms scar tissue, mends fractures. Aids in resisting virus and bacteria infection. Helps in absorption of iron.	Lemons, oranges, acerola cherries, strawberries, papaya, persimmons, kale collard greens, parsley, guavas, turnip greens, most fruits and vegetables.
D	Necessary for bone development regulates amount of calcium and phosphorus in the blood. It's primarily stored in the liver. It can be formed in the body when the direct rays of the sun activate cholesterol in the skin. Too much Vitamin D can cause excess calcium in the blood and tissues.	Sunlight, fish liver oil, egg yolks, organ meat, fatty fishes, milk and milk products
E	Tocopherol. Prevents fats and Vitamin A from breaking down and forming harmful combinations. Helps to heal burns, bruises and external wounds. Unites with oxygen to prevent red blood cells from rupturing. It may help to improve the health of the circulatory system and may help to slow down aging. It also may help to increase fertility and sexual potency.	Margarine, wheat germ, whole grains, eggs, fruits, peanuts and leafy green vegetables.
K	Helps in production of prothrombin, which is necessary for blood clotting. Prevents hemorrhaging.	Oats, wheat, rye, leafy green vegetables alfalfa sprouts and fats

And that's the truth, the whole truth and nothing but the truth about vitamins—what they are for and where you find them. I firmly believe in them and you should too. If you eat the proper foods, you should get all of your proper vitamins and become healthy, happy and live a long, long time.

PROTEIN

If you had to select the one substance in your diet that was of paramount importance that would have to be protein. You may not realize it but between 18 and 20% of your total body weight is protein. In other words if your weight is 100 pounds about 20 pounds of that is protein. About 63% of that goes into your skin, muscles, bone and cartilege. Now get ready for a real shocker. Your hair, your fingernails, your eyes, teeth, heart, lungs, kidneys and nerves are *all* protein. With that in mind you can understand what kind of damage a protein deficient diet can cause. If you engage in a prolonged abstinence from protein—you will die suddenly and permanently.

What exactly is protein? Its a substance composed of about 30 different amino acids. 22 of them are in your body but 8 of them are not and have to be supplied from food. You have to get all eight of them constantly and in exactly the right proportion at exactly the same time. That means you have to find sources of food that supply complete protein.

Another surprise: meat is the worst source of protein contrary to all the steak addicts. The best sources of complete protein are eggs, milk (real milk), soybeans, wheat germ, whole grains and real cereals (not manufactured), cheese (natural not processed), vegetables and dried fruit (watch that high sugar.)

FATS

Fats (contrary to what you may think) are an important part of your diet not only because they are a source of energy but because they act as carriers for the fat-soluble vitamins A, D, E and K. Another important function of fats is their ability to make calcium available to body tissues and bones. Fats also keep your blood, arteries and nerves healthy. If you have dry or scaly skin you probably have a fat deficiency.

Moderation, of course is necessary. Too much fat in your diet can be dangerous. Fat that cannot be fully metabolized (broken down and used) can become toxic. Fats are also necessary to break down cholesterol (which is also a fat).

Fats are composed of two different types of fatty acids. One is called 'saturated' fat—that's usually from animal sources and these kind of fats stay hard at room temperature. The other kind is called 'polyunsaturated' fat—from vegetable sources—which is usually liquid at room temperature.

Two highly important fats (or lipids in your diet are *cholesterol* (the cholesterol in your skin will produce vitamin A when exposed to sunlight) and *lecithin* which is mainly concentrated in the brain and nerve tissues of your body. Highly important, as you can well imagine.

You can obtain fats from milk products, eggs, nuts, seeds, margarine, butter, oils and, of course, meat which is not the best source for fats. In fact, the less meat you have in your diet (if the people of Shangri-La are any example) the longer you can count on living and living well.

CARBOHYDRATES

Here's another area that is misunderstood by most dieters. Certain carbohydrates are vitally necessary in your diet, others can be really harmful. You must understand that if you supply your body with certain carbohydrates your body can use them for immediate energy and body activity and save its protein for building and repair. Otherwise the body will have to break down the protein and use part of it for a carbohydrate. One of the important functions of a carbohydrate is the part it can play in digesting and assimilating foods. It also helps regulate fat and protein metabolism. Incidentally, in case you're wondering, *metabolism* is defined as a total physical and chemical process in which protoplasm is produced, maintained and destroyed and energy is made available for functioning.

All right. So what are carbohydrates anyway? There are three different kinds. There are sugars, starches and cellulose. *Now follow this because it's terribly important.*

SUGARS

There are two kinds of sugars. There are 'single' sugars which you get from all kinds of fruit and from honey. This is the best kind because (a) it's easily digested and (b) because it contains fructose which is the sugar that your brain needs. The other sugar is a 'double' like table sugar which is really bad because it's hard to digest and because of processing has virtually no nutritional value. Stick with fruits and honey you'll be much better off.

STARCHES

They require long digestive action and produce glucose which also is called blood sugar, and is an energy source. Not the best source (fats are the best source of energy). Now the main reason why starches are bad for you is the way most starches are produced in this country. The kind of processing that takes place with white flour and white sugar has eliminated their nutritional value which means you tend to eat *more* to satisfy your natural craving for carbohydrates. The end result is a high rate of diseases that affect the heart and the arteries. Let's face it. White bread, white flour, table sugar, processed 'potato chips' and processed rice are bad for your health. They don't give you proper roughage. That brings us to:

CELLULOSE

That comes from the skins of fruits and vegetables. That's your best source of roughage which regulates the bowels, prevents constipation and creates intestinal activity which prevents the buildup of harmful bacteria in the stomach.

Incidentally, I didn't tell you your best sources for starches. Unrefined wheats and real cereals, nuts, potatoes (eat the skins), root and non-root vegetables, fruits, seeds and honey.

MINERALS

Minerals play an important part in health (and long life) much more so than most people realize. There are about 15 different minerals that are vital to your health. Some of them are familiar to you, but others may not be. Also there are functions of certain minerals that may be unfamiliar to you.

CALCIUM

You probably know that calcium works with phosphorus to build and maintain your bones and teeth. Did you also know that it helps your blood to clot, that it helps maintain the proper balance of acid and alkaline in your blood, that it plays an important part in heartbeat regulation, nerve transmission and muscle contraction? Did you also know that you cannot absorb calcium without the presence of vitamins A, C and D as well as phosphorus? Did you know that calcium when combined with oxalid acid forms a compound which can form into gall stones or kidney stones? (Oxalic acid is found in chocolate, spinach and rhubarb.) You see?

What are your best sources for calcium? Whole sesame seeds, natural (not processed) cheeses like parmesan and swiss. Kelp and other sea weeds, collard greens, almonds, turnip greens, blackstrap molasses and kale. No, Virginia, you *can't* get calcium from pasteurized milk only from *natural* milk.

CHLORINE

Oh, yes, you do need chlorine. Where do you suppose the hydrochloric acid in your stomach comes from? Without it you couldn't digest your food. Chlorine also helps to balance your blood and maintain the proper amounts of acid and alkaline. You get chlorine from ripe tomatoes, celery, lettuce, kelp and spinach. *Don't try to get it from your table salt!*

In fact, the less table salt you use on your food, the better. Excess chlorine has to be excreted and the more you put in your body from table salt the harder your body has to work to get rid of it. Get your salt from natural sources of food.

CHROMIUM

That's right, chromium. Surprised? Well, you better listen because if you don't get your chromium you can get hardening of the arteries or cataracts on your eyes. It's a proven fact that most Americans are chromium deficient because of the high amounts of saturated fats, refined sugars and starches in our diet. Those no-no's run about 60% of the average diet. And that kind of diet depletes the chromium in the body. If you're taking birth control pills you need extra chromium. Are you diabetic? You need extra chromium.

You can get your chromium (along with other good things) from wheat germ, brewer's yeast, nuts, grains, honey, shellfish, chicken, vegetables and fruits.

COBALT

You need cobalt to produce vitamin B12 and for the proper functioning of the red blood cells. You need it every day because there is little or no body storage. The best sources are wheat germ, whole grain cereals, green leafy vegetables, and fruits that have been grown in cobalt-rich soil.

COPPER

It helps form red blood cells and hair pigment (color). It's found in elastic muscle fibers and the covering of nerve fibers. Deficiency is very rare. Best sources are shellfish and organ meats, brewer's yeast, nuts, raisins and prunes. Women need more during pregnancy and menses.

FLUORINE

Not only necessary to prevent tooth decay through the reduction of acid-forming bacteria but also strengthens bones by assisting in the deposition of calcium.

Best sources are tea and seafood.

IODINE

This mineral helps to form thyroxin which controls the normal activity of the thyroid gland. Thyroxin also regulates the body's growth and normal development.

Shellfish offer the best source, much better than table salt.

IRON

This is necessary for the creation of myoglobin (which carries oxygen to muscle tissue) and hemoglobin (which transports oxygen in the blood). There is widespread iron deficiency anemia in this country, particularly in women.

Instead of buying some over-the-counter prescription, get your iron from a natural source like organ meats (liver—all livers—are especially rich in iron), egg yolks too are rich in iron, shellfish, beans (very rich) and green leafy vegetables.

MAGNESIUM

This is one of the most important minerals because it activates more enzymes in the body than any other mineral. It's the primary agent in using fats, proteins, carbohydrates and a number of vitamins and minerals. Magnesium helps to insure proper functions of nerves and muscles (including the heart).

You'll find magnesium in nuts, beans, peanut butter (natural), whole grains, blackstrap molasses, seafood and diary products. Green leafy vegetables are also a good source.

MANGANESE

This is another important activator of enzymes. It's also responsible for normal skeletal development, and maintains blood sugar levels and reproductive processes.

Deficiency in most cases is very rare. You can get your

manganese from nuts, tea, fruits, root vegetables, cereals and grains, green leafy vegetables, spices and condiments.

MOLYBDENUM

Current thinking is that molybdenum is necessary for enzyme functioning. It's stored in the liver and kidneys. It's also supposed to be associated with the functions of vitamin E. It is the least abundant of essential minerals.

You can get your molybdenum from organ meats, grains, cereals, green leafy vegetables, spices and condiments.

PHOSPHORUS

This important mineral plays a major part in almost every chemical reaction in your body and performs more functions than any other mineral. Phosphorus is a major factor in the growth, maintenance and repair of cells, and in energy production. It provides energy for nerve impulses and muscle contractions; it maintains the acid/alkaline balance in the blood, helps to secrete hormones and helps to use fats and fatty-acids. Phosphorus is also involved in the genetic transfer of hereditary characteristics.

You can get phosphorus from wheat germ, brewers yeast, fish, chicken, seeds, dairy products, and powdered skim milk.

POTASSIUM

In the main, potassium works with sodium to form muscle protein and to stimulate nerve impulses for muscle contraction. On its own, potassium helps to convert glucose to glycogen which is easier to store in the body. Potassium also helps maintain the balance of acid/alkalinity in the blood.

You get potassium from green leafy vegetables, like spinach, and from seafood, nuts, fruits and root vegetables.

SELENIUM

There is new thinking about this important mineral. It seems that selenium is an anti-oxidant that can prevent the oxidation of saturated fats in the blood and could thus head off or minimize the possibility of certain diseases like hardening of the arteries. It is also thought that selenium may work with vitamin E in the prevention of certain kinds of cancers. As I said, this is the kind of *thinking* that's going on in laboratories around the country. I have no idea of its validity.

You can get selenium from nuts, seafood, grains, cereals, fruits, organ meats, condiments, spices and natural milk.

SODIUM

Working with potassium, sodium helps maintain balance of acidity/alkalinity of the blood and regulates water balance in your body. It also has an influence on muscular activity. It has been said that sodium aggrevates high blood pressure (see why I want you to cut down on salt?) Get your sodium from natural seafood, chicken, green leafy vegetables and dairy products.

SULFUR

This important mineral helps two B vitamins (thiamin and biotin) to function properly. Sulfur also plays a vital part in the formation (and respiration) of body tissues. If your diet includes a normal amount of protein you'll get all the sulfur your body needs. Here's where you get sulfur from: Fish, eggs, dairy products, nuts and (if you must) meat.

ZINC

That's right, Virginia—*zinc*. It's a very necessary mineral. It's needed to help form enzymes and proteins, helps with your digestion, gets rid of carbon dioxide, helps lower cholesterol levels, and helps with the metabolism of phosphorus.

Zinc deficiency is common among older people and pregnant women. The American diet of refined sugar and flour helps to make this a fairly common deficiency.

You can get your zinc from nuts, meats and shellfish, egg yolks, grains and cereals, spices and condiments.

Current thinking about zinc indicates that it may be of some help in the treatment of schizophrenia (one of the commonest mental illnesses), alcoholism, sexual retardation and Hodgkin's disease. Extra zinc is necessary for women on birth control pills.

Just remember, if you diet properly, with moderation and at proper intervals, you will not only have a healthier body and live much longer—you will find yourself much happier generally and a veritable tiger in bed.

In our next chapter we're going to show you how to Live Longer and Look Younger with simple tuneups and exercises.

WHAT SHOULD YOU WEIGH?

Weight (Indoor Clothing)

Height with Shoes	Small	Medium	Large
4′ 10″	92- 98	96-107	104-119
11″	94-101	98-110	106-122
5′ 0″	96-104	101-113	109-125
1″	99-107	104-116	112-128
2″	102-110	107-119	115-131
3″	105-113	110-122	118-134
4″	108-116	113-126	121-138
5″	111-119	116-130	125-142
6″	114-123	120-135	129-146
7″	118-127	124-139	133-150
8″	122-131	128-143	137-154
9″	126-135	132-147	141-158
10″	130-140	136-151	145-163
11″	134-144	140-155	149-168
6′ 0″	138-140	144-159	153-173

*If you are a woman between 18 and 25 years of age, you should subtract one pound for each year under 25.

WHAT SHOULD YOU WEIGH?

Weight (Indoor Clothing)

Height with Shoes	Small	Medium	Large
5' 2"	112-120	118-129	126-141
3"	115-123	121-133	129-144
4"	118-126	124-136	132-148
5"	121-129	127-139	135-152
6"	124-133	130-143	138-156
7"	128-137	134-147	142-161
8"	132-141	138-152	147-166
9"	136-145	142-156	151-170
10"	140-150	146-160	155-174
11"	144-154	150-165	159-179
6' 0"	148-158	154-170	164-184
1"	152-162	158-175	168-189
2"	156-167	162-180	173-194
3"	160-171	167-185	178-199
4"	164-175	172-190	182-204

While these "new" desirable weight tables are "actuarially sound," and represent average normal patterns of weight, you may still be within a normal weight range for yourself if you are 20% over or 10% under the figures given above. Beyond that range you owe yourself a medical check-up for professional diagnosis and possible assistance in your personal weight-control program.

CHAPTER SIX

HOW TO LIVE LONGER, LOOK YOUNGER

Men have expended infinite ingenuity
in establishing the remote rhythms
of the solar systems and the periodicity
of the comet. They have disdained to
trouble about the simpler task of proving
or unproving the cycles of their own organisms.
HAVELOCK ELLIS

There are two promises that are implicit in the title of this chapter. At first glance, neither of them might seem credible. You've heard it all before and you just don't believe that it's possible to live longer or look younger.

Well, you're wrong. It's not only possible, but it will actually happen to you in at least one respect, before you've finished reading this book. How's that for an outrageous claim? It's true. It will actually happen.

You see I'm talking about *looking* younger. There are a number of ways to look younger without makeup or plastic surgery. One of the simplistic statements in that regard would be simply to tell you to 'get healthy'. That's true. Healthy people do look younger. Now if you start following some of the rather sound advice you've had up till now, in the book, relative to eating properly and eliminating the poisons, the drugs, the alcohols, the caffeins and the cigarettes, you will become much healthier. However you can't possibly get that healthy before you finish reading this book (unless you take several months to read it).

No. I promised you that you can look younger before you finish reading this book and I was assuming that you would take at least a day or two. How can it be done in that short time?

Simply by becoming active. When you are active and extremely interested in everything around you, you can't help becoming vivacious. Which means that your body and your face develop movement that imparts a youthful appearance.

So movement, activity, interest are the keys to looking younger. What about living longer? Well those same three things will give you a longer lease on life because your body will stay in shape, the muscles will regain the tone and temper of youth, and your heart will be given the exercise it needs.

Now before you start moaning and groaning at the thought of exercising, let me say that I hate *most* exercises because they're dull and boring. The exercises that I'm going to tell you about are neither. They're quite easy, extremely beneficial and even I enjoy doing them.

It doesn't matter how old you are. Whether you're 20 or 90 you still need a certain amount of exercise every day. Not the kind of bone-cracking, agonizing exercises that the military personnel go through, but simple, easy-to-do, enjoyable exercise that you can derive immediate benefit from.

Now before we tell you about them, there is something you should remember. Before you start any kind of an exercise program you should have a complete physical checkup. You should also take this book along and let your doctor see the kinds of exercises that we're talking about. He'll probably agree, in most cases, that none of these exercises will hurt you. However, there might be some factor that will preclude your taking some of these suggested exercises. So checkup—and checkout, before you start.

HOW TO TUNE UP YOUR HEART

We're going to start with exercises for your heart because that's the most important muscle in your body and if it's not in good shape, both of us are in trouble.

The best place to start with heart exercises is in the morning when you get out of bed. Belay that. Actually you should start *before* you get out of bed. When you wake up is time to start.

You see, all night long, unless you've been trashing around in a nightmare, your heart has been working at a steady pace. So when you wake up in the morning, you should wake up your heart, too. Here's how:

Stretch like a cat while you're still lying in bed. That's all. Just stretch way out, right down to your toes. Now start clenching and unclenching your fists, very rapidly. That acts like a pump and assists your heart in pumping blood through your system at a much faster rate. That little trick does wonders for your complexion, incidentally. It also tones up all your body muscles in addition to your heart muscle.

Keep up the hand pumping and you'll begin to feel warm, really warm, right down to your toes. Now you're ready for phase two of your early morning tune-up exercises. Swing your feet over the bed and sit up slowly. In that sitting position stretch up to the ceiling, then bring your arms down and parallel with the floor. Hold them straight out and rotate your arms slowly by making a letter "O" in the air with your hands. Stop. Reverse the rotation and make the "O" the other way. Drop your hands and relax.

Now sitting very straight and tall, with your arms relaxed, turn your head slowly to the right until your chin touches your right shoulder. Now rotate your head slowly to the left until your chin touches your left shoulder. Do this three times.

Stand up slowly, all the way up until you're standing on the tip of your toes. Reach up with your hands and try to touch the ceiling (regardless of how far away it is). Bring your hands down slowly until your arms are outstretched and parallel with the floor. Do the rotating trick by making an "O" in the air with your outstretched hands.

Now relax for a moment. Then, after a slow count of 5, tense your stomach muscles *and* your buttock muscles. If you have trouble with your buttock muscle tension, try to imagine that you're holding a half dollar between the cheeks and you don't want it to drop. If you have difficulty in imagining—then actually get a half dollar and see if you can hold it there.

Now do a series of relaxing and tensing (using a count of 10 between each series) then walk slowly to the bathroom.

HOW TO WALK

Incidentally, that's the way you should practice walking. If you deliberately tense and relax your stomach and buttock muscles while walking, you increase the benefits of the exercise. Walking, at any age, is one of the healthiest and simplest of all exercises. There are three factors to be considered:

1. *How* you walk is important. Strolling aimlessly is not exercise walking. When you walk, for exercise, you must walk briskly with purpose and good posture.
2. The *distance* you walk is also important. Determine how far you intend to walk before you start out. Always remember that, in the end, the distance is doubled. You have to walk back again—remember? So if you decide to walk 10 blocks (or half a mile) the actual distance will become 20 blocks (or 1 mile).
3. The last determining factor is your age, or health or a combination of the two. Start out slowly for short distances and gradually, day by day, increase the speed and length of your walking tour. It will, as you continue, get easier and easier because your body will respond to this exercise in a surprisingly short time.

Now when you reach the point where you walk quite rapidly for a considerable distance, you should consider "jogging" which is, in many expert's opinion, the finest form of exercise.

Again, when you start jogging, work up to sustained effort gradually—don't try to become an Olympic star overnight.

After you have been jogging for awhile (and gradually increasing your distance) you will find that you can extend yourself with very little effort to the point where you can begin to indulge in modest cross country jogging. Eventually you may even become one of our army of long distance runners.

The point is that your heart will benefit tremendously from this kind of exercise as long as you do it regularly and as long as you do not do it to extremes. I cannot stress that fact too much. Sustained, regular, modern exercise on a regular basis is healthy and beneficial to your heart. Sudden, violent exercise is dangerous for your heart.

Moderation and regularity are the twin keys to keep in mind if you wish to tune-up your heart and your body each day. Incidentally—what do you do if it rains or snows? Then you walk (or job) in place at home for the same length of time you would do it outside. You will derive exactly the same benefits—so long as you have a supply of fresh air.

CLOTHING

A word about your clothing. Be sure to wear loose fitting clothes that are porous and allow air to circulate about your body. The worst thing you can do is to wear tight clothing or clothing that doesn't allow the skin to breathe. You can wear shoes for walking but not jogging. You should have heavy soled sneakers for jogging to protect the bottom of your feet. Never wear your sneakers without socks. The friction of the inside of your sneakers against the skin can give you blisters that can be quite painful.

When you finish your walking or jogging and return home, it's a good idea to take a mild shower and change your clothes. Notice I said 'mild' shower. Never take a hot shower when you are overheated. Your body is trying to cool you down to normal and by taking a hot shower you are aggravating the situation. On the other hand don't take an ice cold shower, you could give yourself a violent shock because the sudden cold will cause your blood vessels to contract and send your blood pressure sky high and you know how dangerous that can be.

I know—you have a friend that takes ice cold showers every morning and he's in the pink of health. Fine. Maybe he is and maybe he isn't. Do you know exactly what kind of condition you're in right now? Would you like to find out? Then do this:

1. Stand up, take a deep breath, exhale fully, then relax.
2. Close your eyes, place your hands on your hips.
3. Now, slowly and carefully, lift one foot off the ground.
4. Try to maintain your balance in that position while you count, "One locomotive, Two locomotives, etc. until you reach "Twenty locomotives". If you did it slowly and deliberately, you have reached at least 20 seconds time.

Now the *easier* it was to maintain your balance (with your eyes closed) for that full 20 seconds—the better your general physical condition. The more difficult it was, the lower the mark you give yourself (and the more reason for starting your exercise program immediately).

TAKE YOUR PULSE

Here's another way to check yourself. Take your own pulse. It's not difficult. All you need is a watch or a clock with a sweep second hand that's easy to see. What you are going to do is count the number of times your heart beats in a one minute period. However, instead of taking your pulse for a full minute, your best bet is to take it for 6 seconds—count the number of times your heart beats in that 6 second period and then multiply that number by 10. Six times ten is sixty. So if your heart beats 9 times in that 6 seconds, your heart beats 90 times in a minute.

Here's how you take your own pulse. Use your right or left forefinger (never your thumb because it has a beat of its own that will confuse you) and locate a little hollow just below your wristbone (with the palm of your hand facing you). Just insert your forefinger in that little hollow and you will feel a distinct pulse that's easy to count. All you have to do is count the number of pulses or beats within a 6 second period and then multiply that number by 10.

A pulse rate between 60 and 85 beats per minute is normal, when resting. A good idea would be to write down the pulse rate and place the date next to it. Later, when you start your exercise program, you can begin to record your pulse rate, day by day, and you will begin to see the change that takes place as you get stronger and healthier.

Now here is a special test that you can try later on, when you feel that you're really in shape. I mean that. *Do not try this test unless you feel that you're in pretty good physical condition.* If you think you are, here's how it's done.

It requires that you use a platform that is 15 to 20 inches high. If you haven't got one and you have access to stairs then do this exercise *at the bottom of the stairs*—using the distance of the first two steps (about 18 inches).

Place one foot on the second step, then step up and back down, with the other foot, 30 times in one minute. Then take your pulse. Wait a minute, take it again. Wait another minute and take it again. Wait one more minute and take it a final time. Now *add* the first pulse (highest) with the lowest pulse rate following that. Then check that figure against this table:

Less than 132	Excellent
133 to 150	Very Good
151 to 170	Good
171 to 198	Fair
199 and higher	Poor

This test, incidentally, is part of the test program given under the auspices of the President's Council on Physical Fitness. The idea is that there should not be too much difference (after a few minutes rest) in the pulse rate when activated and the pulse rate when inactive. There is, of course, a marked difference immediately after strong physical effort, but the heart should return to a fairly normal beat very shortly.

Please remember, if you decide to take this test, to stop if you experience dizziness or shortness of breath. It is a bit strenuous, particularly if you haven't been exercising for quite a while. That's one of the reasons why I stressed the fact that you should do it at the *bottom* of the stairs.

If you do take the test, write down the results and the date. Then, after you've been on your regular xercise program for a couple of weeks—take the test again and notice the big difference in the results.

Just keep the two factors in mind when you start your physical fitness program. Moderation and regularity. Do all your exercises in moderation and do them regularly every day without fail, rain or shine.

BENEFITS

Regardless of your age, whether you are young, middle aged or old, if you haven't been exercising regularly, please start slowly and work up gradually. Intensity is not as important as the length of time you spend. Think of it in terms of consecutive minutes. The most beneficial results of the increased oxygen in your lungs and the increased circulation of your blood will take place after 6 consecutive minutes. In this time you will have reached the light 'panting stage'—plus a little light perspiration. Your body, at this point, will be alive with increased vigor and vitality and you should feel quite good. You will feel good physically and good mentally (because you accomplished what you set out to do) and both of those 'good' feelings are beneficial.

There are interesting benefits you will become aware of as you progress with your physical fitness program. One is that tension and anxiety will lessen considerably.

That decrease in tension and anxiety will help you with the other part of your program. It will help you to begin to eliminate your dependency on cigarettes, alcohol, sleeping pills, tranquilizers, etc. It will also help you to establish sensible eating habits. Now, as your dietary habits improve your physical rehabilitation will improve. This, in turn, will increase the benefits of your exercise and your health will begin to improve at a faster and faster rate.

Your most immediate and noticeable result will be the tremendous improvement in your *mental* outlook. Your mind will become alive in a way that will startle you. Your horizons will begin to broaden; each thing you see and come in contact with will take on a fresh new meaning. Colors will be more vivid than you have ever seen them. Everything you do will provide you with keen enjoyment and deep pleasure.

This begins to happen almost from the moment you make your decision to live longer, look younger and enjoy life. You will find that you begin to look for new and different ways to increase your capacity for exercise. Taking out the garbage is no longer a chore—it's a chance to exrcise. You'll find yourself skipping the elevator ride and choosing to walk up the stairs instead. If you're on the golf course you'll decide to leave the cart and walk around the 18 holes instead.

Another dramatic difference is the increased agility you will discover. Your coordination will improve markedly. So will your posture (which will cause many people to remark how well you look without realizing why). Most of all, your energy will, after a time, seem to be almost endless. That will be a combination result—from a better diet and from healthy exercise. You will be deriving all of the benefits of a healthy body and an active interested mentality.

ISOMETRICS

One of the most popular forms of exercise is Isometrics because it requires no equipment, can be done anywhere by anyone at any age. The isometric exercises involve muscular stress for short periods of time. The simplest demonstration is to open your left hand, make a fist with your right hand and then press your fist against the palm of your left hand as hard as you can. At the same time resist the pressure with your left arm as hard as you can. Do this with all your strength for a count of 10 and then relax. Reverse your hands. Make a fist of your left hand and try to press it against the palm of your right hand. Press and resist as hard as you can for a slow count of ten and relax. Muscular tension and then relaxation. That's all there is to it. There are a variety of different exercises. However, isometrics, according to some authorities, is not good for people with bad hearts because it involves effort that markedly affects the heart, lungs and blood vessels. So before you try any of these isometric exercises, check it out with your doctor if you have a heart condition.

Again, as we said before, moderation and regularity are the keynotes. Start out gradually and work up to higher intensities as your muscles become tuned up and more powerful.

ISOMETRIC EXERCISE 1

Interlock your fingers, thumbs upward. Place your palms against your forehead. Push against your head at the same time your head pushes against your palms. Do this exercise for a count of five slow 'locomotives' (one locomotive, two locomotives, etc.). Then, relax for 2 minutes.

ISOMETRIC EXERCISE NO. 2

Sit on the floor in an open doorway. Stretch out your legs with your feet in the center of the doorway. Now open your legs and press against the sides of the doorway as though you intended to widen the doorway with the pressure. Keep pressing for 6 seconds (six locomotives) then stop and relax.

ISOMETRIC EXERCISE NO. 3

Stand at the open doorway with your hands braced against the doorframe. Set yourself so that your right foot is forward and then press against the doorframe for 5 seconds. Relax for a count of 10 and then put your left foot forward and press against the doorframe for 5 seconds. Relax and rest.

ISOMETRIC EXERCISE NO. 4

Raise your arms to your shoulders height. Hold them straight out and parallel to the floor. Now, keeping your upper arms at shoulder height, bend your arms at elbow, curl the fingers of your hands and lock them together. Now try to pull them apart for a slow count of 10. Relax for 2 minutes.

ISOMETRIC EXERCISE NO. 5

(While driving your car)
1. Squeeze the steering wheel as tightly as you can for 5 seconds.
2. Tense the upper muscles of your legs for 5 seconds.
3. Make a fist of your toes for 5 seconds.
4. Tense your stomach muscles for 5 seconds.

Relax and let 2 minutes pass between each of these exercises. They will keep your muscles toned during a long ride and help to keep you alert.

YOGA

Now we are going to explore some of the exercises that have come to the western world from ancient eastern world. You have probably heard of Yoga. It is not, as many people believe, a religious or mystical cult but rather an ancient Hindu system that is concerned with bringing the body to perfect pitch and harmony. We are not suggesting that you become an adept and reach the peak of astonishing control that most of the serious practitioners of the art achieve. We are going to employ certain exercises to restore your body to its natural, healthy state.

There are three main avenues within Yoga—ASANA, which is concerned with posture, PRANAYAMA which is concerned with breath control and MEDITATION which is achievement of the Alpha State (slower brain waves).

We are going to concentrate our efforts on HATHA YOGA which is considered as the initial purification and preparation for all of the higher forms of Yoga. In these exercises you will find that there is emphasis on stretching and flexibility. I can promise you that these exercises, if regularly pursued, will free you forever of most of your muscular pains and most particularly, your back pain problems will disappear like magic unless, of course, they are caused by something other than bad posture or weak and strained muscles.

RELAXATION

Place a quilt or a pair of blankets on the floor, remove your shoes and be certain that none of your clothing is tight. In fact, the less clothes you wear the better. Now lie down, stretch out, then let go and completely relax. Let your head fall to one side. This simple position is called SAVASANA. Just relax and try to picture this scene in your mind:

You are lying on a hill side in the hot sun, surrounded by a mass of fragrant flowers. The only sound is the soft sighing of the warm breeze and you're at complete peace with yourself and the world. You haven't a care in the world. You don't have to be anywhere, do anything, but just lie there and enjoy this utterly peaceful and relaxing time.

Would you prefer the soft white sands of the seashore with the muffled roar of the surf and a hot sun beating down on you, cooled by the fragrant salt air breeze passing over you?

Or would you rather be indoors in a luxurious bedroom, in a magnificent feather bed, lying upon satin sheets, with the faint, delicious odors of tantalizing perfume wafting over you and you are neither awake or asleep—just drifting without a care in the world?

Just pick one of the scenes, or write up your own scenario as long as it pleases and relaxes you. The main point is that this gentle and relaxing exercise offers you and your body more health and well being than you could possibly imagine.

STRETCHING EXERCISES

1. Now bring your legs together. Bring your hands together and interlock the fingers. Now, with the palms facing each other, slowly bring your hands (hands still interlocked) high above your head. High as you can reach. Now, slowly and gently, with your fingers still interlocked, turn your palms outward as far as they will go. You will feel an amazing stretch take place in your arms, ribs and in your back muscles.
Now slowly return to your original position, with your arms down, resting on your body and completely relax.
2. Stretch up your arms again as you did the first time, but now, in addition, point your toes and push them against an imaginary wall, directly in front of your toes. Now you should feel the pull in your legs, arms and shoulders.

Remember these exercies and do them gently, each morning when you awaken. Really stretch, and, at the same time, open your mouth and yawn like a cat. You'll be astonished at what a difference this is going to make in a relatively short time.

RHYTHMIC ROCKING EXERCISE

Sit down on the floor and draw up your knees with your fingers behind your knees. Keep your body (torso) and your head erect. Now slowly let your body (still keeping your hands in position) roll gently backwards until your legs are above your face and your head is reting on the floor. Then rock gently forward again until youregain your original position. As you continue doing this you will become more and more proficient until you can do it easily and continuously with very little effort. In some respects the benefits of this exercise resemble those derived from chiropractic admustment of the spine. You will derive considerable calmness and at the same time, energy will be released. Above all, this simple exercise will give you extraordinary pleasure as you become more and more proficient in its execution.

YOGAMUDRA

Now here is an excellent exercise which is an important Asana for inner purification. At the same time it's an amazing antidote for constipation. Here's how you do it.

1. Sit on the floor in a 'tailor fashion' position. Now make your hands into fists and place a fist on either side of your navel. Then bend forward and touch your head to the floor (or as close as you can come at first). Now as you move backwards and forward slowly and gently. As you do so, your fists will massage your inner organs.

NOTE: If you drink 6 to 10 glasses of water daily not only will you eliminate constipation, but you will improve your body functions quite noticeably.

Perhaps you may have wondered (if you are familiar with Yoga) why I have not mentioned the graceful and highly beneficial Lotus Position. You should remember that it is a most difficult position to assume until your body has come to acquire more suppleness with repeated exercise.

When you do reach that advanced state and wish to assume the Lotus Position, your hands will be behind your back and as you bend forward and touch your head to the floor, your heels will massage your inner organs as your clenched fists do in the simpler position shown before.

SOME EASY TUNE-UP EXERCISES

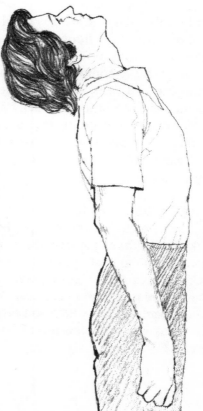

1. THE NECK STRETCH
Standing erect, hands at your sides, relaxed, you point your chin at the ceiling. Hold it in that position for a slow count of 5. Then slowly rotate your chin, clockwise, until your chin is in the original (pointed towards ceiling) position. Repeat this exercise 5 times in the beginning, then increase the number of times by 2 each day until you reach 15 times.

2. THE WINDMILL

Standing erect, hands at your sides, slowly raise your arms to shoulder level, parallel to the floor. Now slowly rotate your arms in the widest circle you can achieve comfortably. Continue this exercise until you have made 10 continuous revolutions. Each day, when you do this exercise, increase the number of revolutions by 5 until you reach a maximum of 60 revolutions at a single exercise.

3. BACK BEND STRETCH

Standing erect, hands on hips, bend backward as far as you can, then come forward to a rest position. Bend backward again. Repeat this exercise 5 times. Increase 2 times each day. You should reach a point where you can do this easily and rhythmically 5 to 15 times.

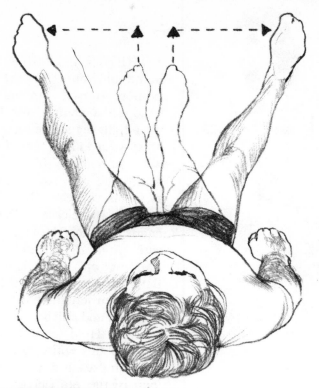

4. ABDOMINAL STRETCH

Lie on your back with your hands at your sides. Your feet should be approximately twelve inches apart. Now, with your legs straight, lift your feet six inches from the floor. Hold that position for a count of 5. Then still holding your feet 6 inches from the floor, spread your legs as far as you can and hold them at that position for a count of 5, then return your feet to a point 12 inches apart (still 6 inches off the floor) and hold for a count of 5, then raise your feet approximately 6 inches more, hold for a count of 5, then return to original position, 6 inches above the floor, hold for a count of 5 and then return them to the floor and relax. Now do the entire exercise in a rhythmic pattern.

1. Up to 6 inches, hold to 5 then
2. Spread your legs and hold till 5 then
3. Bring back your feet to 12 inches apart, hold for 5 then
4. Raise your feet another six inches and hold for 5, then
5. Down to original position and hold for 5 then down to floor.

Repeat the entire 5 part exercise 5 times. Each time you do this exercise, increase the number of complete points by 1 until you can do the exercise 10 times without effort.

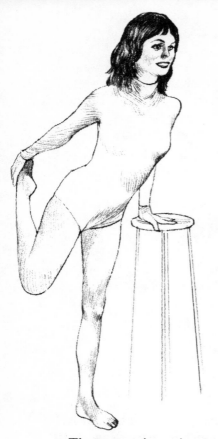

5. THIGH EXTENSION

Stand on your left foot and support yourself with your left hand on a chair. Now bend your right leg at the knee and grasp your ankle (behind you) with your right hand. Now gently pull your right leg back as far as you can. Hold for a count of 10, release and switch hands and leg. Hold a chair with your right hand while standing on your right leg. Bend your left leg at the knee, grasp your left ankle with your left hand and pull back as far as possible. Hold for a count of ten. Do this entire exercise 5 times and each day you do it increase the total (left and right legs) by 1 until you reach 10 complete exercises easily.

These exercises, simple as they are, offer you two types of rewards. The first is long term and that is extended life span. The second reward is suppleness, improved muscle tone, greater vigor, increased circulation, a better appetite and an increased interest in every kind of mental and physical pleasure including sex.

WORD OF WARNING

Great as the rewards are, there is a tendency to believe that 'more is better' and to some extent this is true. However, there is also the danger that sudden intensive effort can prove to be a dangerous adventure.

Shoveling snow is an excellent example. To some people this might seem to be a good opportunity to engage in exercise and at the same time accomplish something useful. *Wrong*. The majority of medical authorities agree that shoveling snow is a task that should be reserved for those in excellent physical condition. The N.Y. Medical Journal published an article in which the author stated, *"Only a person who walks one mile continuously per day should shovel snow."*

If you don't walk that daily mile, or if you are not absolutely certain that you are in peak physical condition, don't shovel snow. Shoveling snow places a great strain on the heart, particularly when the weather is extremely cold. In fact, strenuous exercise should be avoided during any extreme weather condition, hot or cold because extremes of heat and cold place an extra burden on your physical system which must work very hard to maintain your normal body temperatures.

Again, I will repeat the two important keys to all exercising—moderation and regularity. If you use common sense and do not overdo the intensity of your exercises; if you do your exercises faithfull and regularly, you will derive maximum benefit from them.

There is a definite relationship between your mental and physical health and the outward look you present to the world. When you look well, people respond to that factor. In responding to it they make you aware of how well you look. This, in turn, makes you feel even better.

This sort of 'positive feedback' effect works at any age. It provides you with that extra lift that can carry you through the worst days so that regardless of the crisis you are relaxed and confident while all around you chaos reigns.

COMPLEXION

Nothing in this world makes a man or woman feel better than the knowledge that they have healthy, glowing complexion. This is no accident. It's a direct result of proper nutrition, healthy exercise, sufficient natural sleep and a keen and positive mental outlook. All these things can be achieved. However there are certain other factors that can help, as well.

FACTS ABOUT PERSPIRATION

If you listen to (and believe) the many radio and TV commercials that deal with perspiration, you might assume that perspiration is an 'evil' that must be avoided at all costs. Wrong. Perspiration is a natural and vital function that is necessary to our health and well being. The primary function of perspiration is to reduce our body temperature to safe and normal limits. That's the reason why we have pores in our skin. Our skin must be able to breathe and perspire or we would die.

There are two 'evils' according to the advertising hucksters. One is perspiration stains on our clothing and the other is B.O. the terrible Body Odor dragon that we must avoid at all costs. How do we avoid it? *By using their products naturally.*

Wrong again. Products that prevent you from perspiring can be dangerous. Products that neutralize odors but do not prevent perspiration are better but not much.

Let's take them in the following order:

1. BODY ODOR
2. PERSPIRATION

and see if there isn't a natural way to deal with both of these 'problems' as they relate to our modern society.

BODY ODOR

There are two key places where body odor is most noticeable: Under your armpits and in the area around your genitals. Naturally cleanliness is extremely important. Not just by taking showers but by wearing fresh clothes. Most people who are sensitive to the possibility of body odor do take these common sense precautions—*and they still have body odor.* That's because they have only approached the secondary cause of body odor. The primary cause is your diet. You see perspiration is composed of water, salt and some waste material. Your diet will determine the intensity of odor. If you eat a great deal of beef there is a strong possibility that you will have a strong body odor. If you switch from meat (a good idea, incidentally) to another form of protein you might be surprised at the difference in your body odor. Everyone exudes some body odor—some people's body odor is quite fragrant and delightful—other are noxious. You can change the quality of yours by the way you eat. Try it and see what a difference it makes.

PERSPIRATION

If we become overheated we will perspire. That's a fact of life. How do we become overheated? Sometimes through exertion like sustained exercise which increases our body temperature and sometimes through stress induced by fear or anger. We can also perspire freely during sexual intercourse.

The fact is we don't mind perspiring when we exercise or when we are having sex, it's *social* perspiring that worries us.

Oddly enough worrying about perspiring can cause you to perspire, so the first thing to do is stop worrying about it. As your health improves and your physical and mental condition improves you will find that you worry much less and, at the same time, you perspire less.

One of the facts of life is that most anti-perspirants will work because you have confidence that they will keep you 'cool and dry'. It's much the same effect as the belief in aspirin. They work because you believe that they will work.

Now if you can begin to generate the same belief in yourself as you have in these patent drugs, then you will not only save money but you will be far healthier. Many people perspire but do not stain their clothes. Why? Because of their *diet*. Their perspiration is light and it's free of the kind of waste products that stain. Those stain factors come straight from your diet.

You will find, as you proceed with your program of proper nutrition and exercise that many of the problems you have faced in the past will rapidly disappear. Your diet has a great deal to do with your complexion. You will not get the *'skin you love to touch'* from soap and water alone—you will get it when you start to eat properly. Bumps and blemishes will disappear.

ABOUT SOAP

Soap is soap regardless of the advertising claims. The prime function of soap is to assist in the removal of the dead skin that continually appears on the surface of your regular epidermis. That's it—period. If you want a different shape or exotic perfumes in your soap it will cost you more. You will not derive any additional benefits from that more expensive soap. It will not make your skin 'healthier' or more attractive. It will just cost you more money.

A good idea is to wash your skin at night with soap and water because this allows your skin to recover its natural acidity during the night. In the morning use the 'swedish' trick of soaking a clean washcloth in very hot water then wringing it almost dry and applying the hot washcloth to your face gently.

You must just be certain that you wring it out carefully. Gently clean your eyes, face, neck and ears with this hot washcloth. It invigorates the skin and gives you a natural glow. Incidentally always do this with a clean, fresh washcloth. Do not use a wash cloth *more than once* on your face because it picks up a lot of dirt and germs while it's drying out. If you want to avoid this and don't want to increase your washload, then wash the wash cloth thoroughly in hot water and soap before using it. Many skin infections can be caused by dirty washcloths. Also dirty pillowslips. Never take a nap on the couch and use the regular couch pillows. They're dirtier than you can imagine. If you perspire then the dirt can work into your pores and cause all sorts of trouble.

GETTING THAT RICH TAN

Sunlight is vital to good health. In addition to producing vitamin A (interaction of ultraviolet rays with cholesterol in your skin) the rays also help your body to assimilate other vitamins. However, there is a danger in excess exposure to strong sunlight. Beware of the dangers that may come when you try to get a dark tan. Skin cancer has been connected to excessive sun exposure. Not immediately—but later in life. Also you can wind up with a skin like fine old leather.

So again—moderation is the key note. Avoid overexposure particularly when you're at the sea shore or out on a boat. The reflective qualities of water can give you a painful burn.

It would be a wise idea to use sunscreen lotions (as opposed to sun tan lotions) because the sunscreen lotions block about 25% of the ultra-violet rays. However, just because you're covered with these sunscreen lotions don't think that you can overdo the exposure. 25% is not 100%—so prolonged exposure *even with the screen* can add up to just as harmful effect.

SLEEPING IN THE RAW

Winter or summer the best idea is to sleep nude and permit your body to have the freedom it doesn't have during the day. It will also allow a period of time when your body can breathe freely, which is very important.

Another benefit is the possibility that it may enhance your sex life which is not only healthy—it's good for your heart! That's a proven fact, you know. Good, healthy sex is an excellent exercise for the heart and a tonic for the mind and body. So do indulge—if only for the sake of your health.

ALLERGIES

Many allergies (not all, by any means) are now being viewed as products of the *mind* rather than of the body. Many carefully controlled research programs have demonstrated that it is often the *belief* in the presence of certain substances that triggers the allergy symptoms. For example, people who are 'allergic' to certain flowers have, upon entering a room with a bouquet of these particular flowers, immediately exhibited symptoms of allergenic reaction—sneezing, running eyes, etc.

They have been astonished when shown that the flowers were artificial and made out of paper. In many cases these 'allergies' disappeared and never re-occurred.

However, if you should suddenly experience a number of peculiar reactions when you start to use a new product like a cleanser or furniture polish (or new cosmetics) stop using it immediately and check with your family doctor. Skin rashes or excessive itching should be checked immediately to determine the cause. If could be something you've eaten or some substance that you are now exposed to. The same holds true of any medication that you might be taking for the first time. It doesn't necessarily mean that you have an allergy—it might just be an incompatibility with the particular drug. Be sure— check it out with your doctor.

COSMETICS

We Americans spend in the neighborhood of 8 BILLION dollars every year on cosmetics. That figure includes men and women. Yes, Virginia, more and more *men* are using cosmetics these days. My feeling about cosmetics is very simple. There is nothing more attractive in a man or woman than a natural, healthy complexion. Very few cosmetics do more than hide your skin. If you have scars or birthmarks that are unpleasant to you, then by all means use cosmetics to hide them, but if you have a natural healthy skin, it's a shame to cover it up and prevent it from breathing properly.

However, little that I say in this regard will make any difference to you—you're still going to use cosmetics. So do this, at least. Wash it all off before going to sleep at night. This will give your skin at at least a fighting chance to recover while you're sleeping. Be especially careful about eye makeup because there have been a number of cases where people suffered severe eye damage from certain eye makeups.

EYEDROPS

This nonsense about 'red' eyes and the drops that can give you clear white eyes would be ludicrous if it wasn't that there are certain dangers in it. You will only get temporary relief from these drops. The red will come back stronger than ever. Most 'red' eyes come from lack of sleep, too much liquor and cigarettes and a combination of all three. Some red eyes are the signal of a disease and should be checked by your doctor. The best thing for your red eyes is sleep, lots of fresh water, eliminating liquor and cigarettes for a while, or entirely.

The less junk you put in your eyes the better. If you want to wash your eyes thoroughly—work up a good cry for yourself, watch a sad movie or read a sad book or just feel sorry for yourself for a little while. The tears you produce are free and they're the best eyewash you can get.

ABOUT YOUR HAIR

One of the major concerns, of both men and women, down through the ages, has been a fear of becoming bald. Julius Caesar, it is said, wore his laurel leaves constantly, not so much as a crown, but to hide his baldness. Queen Elizabeth (the first) was said to be bald as a billiard ball and wore a fiery red wig. Her arch rival, Mary Queen of Scots, it is alleged, stunned the executioner who had cut off her head. When he bent down and attempted to lift the head to show to the spectators (a grisly custom) he was astonished to find that he had her wig in his hand. The severed head rolled over and stared at him with a mirthless grin.

We are, in this day and age, it would seem, more afraid of losing our hair than of growing old. We seem to equate baldness with old age and a loss of 'sex appeal' even though a number of movie and television stars have demonstrated that there is still plenty of charisma in a bald or shaven head.

Regardless of that fact, there is a booming business in wigs, toupes, hair transplants and hair weaving, not to mention the many 'institutes' that cater to 'hair treatment'.

There are certain basic facts that you must face with regard to hair and how to take care of your hair. Forget about baldness. You are either going to be bald or you are not. There's nothing you can do about it short of hair transplants. If you have a head of hair, take care of it properly and chances are you will go through your entire life with 80% of it intact.

Beautiful hair is dependent upon health. Your health and your hair's health. Now, in the chapter about vitamins we mentioned all of the foods that you need to stay healthy. Stay healthy and it's a good bet your hair will be healthy. It only needs a clean scalp and a continuous nourishment from a strong circulation of good, rich blood. (Also B complex each day helps.)

SCALP MASSAGE

Just as healthy teeth are dependent upon healthy gums, so healthy hair is dependent upon a healthy scalp. You massage your gums every day (or should) and you should massage your scalp every day (or should). Here's how:

Place your thumbs back of your ears and spread the fingers of each hand over the fore part of your scalp. Then rotate the scalp under your fingers. Make sure that it's your scalp that's rotating, not your fingers. Do not scrub your scalp with your fingers. You are trying to maintain a loose scalp to insure proper circulation of the blood through the fatty tissue.

Now press your fingers down and make your scalp move. A tight scalp means you haven't been massaging it enough. Do it at least once each day. Twice (once in the morning and once at night is even better). You want that scalp to be loose.

You should also brush your hair every morning and every night. Always brush under the hair and upward (to lift the scalp and to brush the natural oils into the hair and to give it a natural shine. Be sure the brush has natural bristles (not nylon which can scratch your scalp) and be sure to clean the brush frequently to remove dust, flakes and lint. Never—repeat *never*—use anybody else's brush or comb. Your body bacteria is different and you don't know what kind of scalp disease the other people have. Wash your combs and brushes frequently.

WASHING YOUR HAIR

You must keep your hair clean. If you live in a dirty city and do not wear a hat, your hair will collect a lot of dirt—so will your scalp. You should wash more frequently than your country cousin who lives in a less polluted environment.

The question of 'which shampoo" is an important one. You are bombarded endlessly with TV commercials about this and that shampoo. Your best bet is to visit a really good beauty parlor or a hair care center. They will examine your hair and recommend the type of shampoo and conditioner you need.

Yes, you do need a conditioner because after you have shampooed your hair it's out of balance. The proper conditioner can restore the balance until your body restores it.

Never scrub your hair with a towel after you've washed it. You can really damage it that way. Lower your head, smooth out all the water you can *gently* but firmly. Then encase your hair in a towel and blot it carefully, then wrap the towel around your head and let it dry for a while. Then lower your head and brush it semi-dry. Then either dry it with *gentle* heat or let it dry.

Brush it again when it's dry. It's good for your scalp and it's good for your hair. Remember, brush from the scalp out. If you bend your head while brushing you promote circulation to the scalp which is also helpful.

CUTTING YOUR HAIR

Never have your hair cut when the moon is full. Laugh if you want to, but remember that a lot of successful farmers all over the world never plant during a full moon. They only plant when the new moon begins. They believe that as the moon grows it has a progressively stronger effect on growing things. They also believe that as the full moon weakens it has a bad effect on growing things. It's your hair. Do what you want but remember—it can't hurt to try it. And it might help.

DANDRUFF

Everyone has dandruff—if you're referring to the skin that flakes off from your scalp. After all, skin flakes off all over your body every day—why shouldn't it flake off from your scalp?

However, excessive flaking could be a sign of the onset of a disease of the scalp. Visit a licensed dermatologist. If, after an examination, your dermatologist prescribes medication, use it. Do NOT try to medicate yourself with the nostrums that are advertised on TV. You could cause harm besides throwing your money away.

YOUR FEET

Very few people (outside of shoe salesmen or foot doctors) ever talk about your feet. They're important. You only have one pair to last you an entire lifetime which—if you follow the tips in this book—may be a lot longer than you think. So it would seem that it's a sound idea to take care of your feet.

The first requirement is to keep them clean. You should wash and soak them every day by themselves. Not just in the shower where they get a lick and a promise. But they should be massaged every night before you go to sleep. You should exercise them by making fists (try it, you'll be surprised how adept you can get at making a fist with your feet).

Be sure the shoes you buy fit properly. Stop trying to shove your feet into Cinderella's slipper. Get the proper size and support you need. And buy several pairs of shoes at one time so that you have plenty of changes. Never wear the same pair of shoes each day. It's bad for your feet and its bad for your shoes. Both your feet and your shoes will last longer if you change your shoes regularly.

Same with socks. If possible try not to wear the same socks or stockings or panty hose all day. Change at least once, if possible twice a day. Your feet will feel much better for it. Now I know I may raise some eyebrows with this next statement:

Please do not wear socks to bed. Let your feet breathe during the night. Also, if you wear support stockings, take them off at your earliest opportunity. If you sit for any length of time your support stockings can cut off circulation.

Cut your toenails and if you develop ingrown toenails have them taken care of immediately. Do not try to do it yourself—you'll only make matters worse and, if you're not careful, you can wind up with a nasty infection.

And that brings us to a summation relative to our basic promise to you that we would show you ways to live longer and look younger. I think that we have amply demonstrated that if you feed your body properly and eliminate the poison drugs, alcohol, cigarettes, sleeping pills and tranquilizers; if you exercise in moderation and with regularity; if you cleanse your body and eliminate deodorants, anti-perspirants, cosmetics and laxatives; if you do all these things, that you will most certainly live longer and look younger.

Now, in our next chapter we're going to talk about *enjoying* that longer life. We're going to talk about sexual activity and long life. We're going to show you *why sex is good for you* and can actually prolong your life.

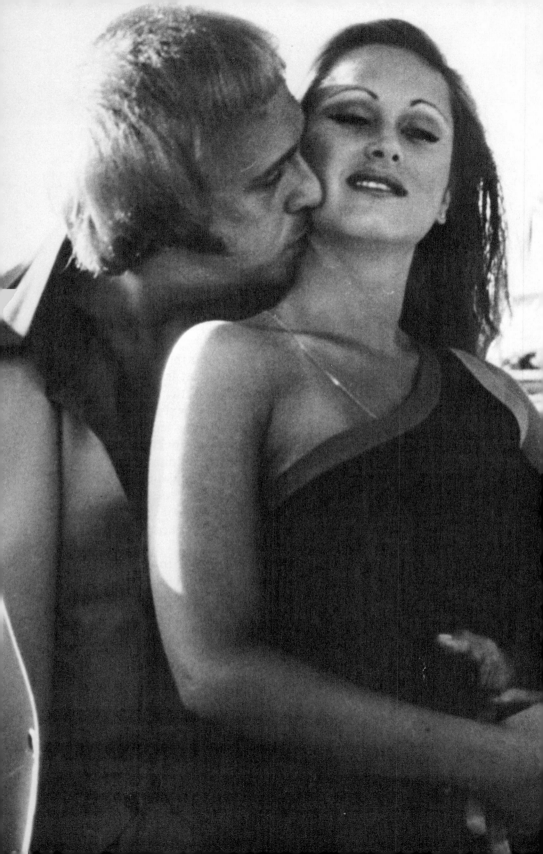

CHAPTER SEVEN
SEXUAL ACTIVITY AND LONG LIFE

When Time and all his tricks
have done their worst
Still will I hold you dear
and him accurst.
                    EDNA ST. VINCENT MILLAY

When medical authorities announced that sexual activity was good for your heart—even for those with heart trouble—it was, to say the least, a startling announcement. It was particularly so for those who had regretfully given up the delight and enjoyment they derived from sexual activity.

When further studies proved that there was a definite relationship between sexual activity and a longer life span that news was even more startling than the earlier announcement. Now, for the first time, people began to realize that by eliminating sex from their lives they were actually shortening their lives. Strangely enough, the majority of people who had eliminated sex were convinced that it was wrong to stop having sex. They could not quite convince themselves that something as basic and natural as the sex act could possibly be bad.

It's not bad for you. It never has been. What has been bad was the *guilt* associated with sex. That's bad for you. Very bad and the ridiculous part is that you never should have been made to feel guilty in the first place. To make someone feel guilty about sexual desires is as insane as to make someone feel guilty about breathing. Both are essential to continued life. Take either one of them away and death is sure to follow.

We now know that another idiotic notion is that 'you get too old for sex'. Strangely enough, even though everyone still had the old urges, very few people ever talked about it. They just assumed that there was something wrong with them. Just them. No one else. That was obvious because no one talked about it. Ergo—each person thought they were the only one with this 'unnatural desire' and therefore thought they were depraved or a freak of some kind.

Well that sort of guilt can now be eliminated forever.

Now let's look at some of the facts about human sexuality and long life. We already know that sexual activity is good for the heart and naturally the better your heart is, the longer it's going to beat. That much is certain. There must be more to it than that. There certainly is. The key is *hormone production.*

Studies have shown that if you *decrease* hormone production rapid aging begins to take place and an early death is certain. If the hormone production is *increased* then aging is actually reversed and a much longer life span is the end result (if all other factors are also present. Factors such as we have talked about in the previous chapter.)

Castrated males (physically or mentally) have early deaths.

Females, when they enter menopause, age rapidly and can die early deaths.

Medical intervention in the form of injections of the male hormone (testosterone) have produced remarkable rejuvenation. However, much of that was discontinued due to unfortunate side effects.

Females have been luckier in that estrogen (female hormone) therapy has slowed and, in some cases, reversed aging and a longer life expectancy was produced.

There is a perfectly natural way to increase hormone (male) production and that's through regular sexual intercourse. There is also a correlation in the well being of a female who enjoys sexual intercourse on a regular basis. It's a mental and physical boost and, of course, excellent for the heart.

So now, for the first time, we have clear evidence that if you have an active and enjoyable sex life, you will not only be much healthier but your life expectancy will be increased immeasurably. It seems that there couldn't be a happier state of affairs.

Unfortunately we do not have 'a happier state of affairs.'
For many different reasons.

SIDELIGHTS ON SEX

In spite of the widespread dissemination of information about sex, sexual intercourse, sexual attitudes and sex therapy, there is probably more ignorance about sex than you would ever imagine. Take your closest friends, for example. You must know them fairly well. Try to imagine what their reaction would be if they were guests in your home for an evening and someone mentioned the subject of 'sex'.

Now go a step further. What do you suppose their reaction would be if the term 'sexual intercourse' were used in the general conversation? What would your reaction be? Would you be embarrassed?

Without reference to the knowledge you now have with respect to sex and old age, what would your normal reactions be to the following statements if you heard them at a party:

1. **Sex isn't important after 70**
2. **Older men are impotent; they have no erections**
3. **Women lose sexual desire after menopause**

Would you have believed those three statements? If you didn't believe them, would you have argued about them? Do you think that there's something 'not quite right' about a woman of 80 deciding to marry a man of 90? Are you embarrassed when you hear that they are both eager for sex?

While you're thinking about those questions let me tell you about how the majority of people feel about them. In the main most people believe that the items 1., 2. and 3. are true. Most people are embarrassed by the idea of two 'older' people marrying and looking forward to sexual relations.

Most people believe that 'sex' is something that only concerns 'younger people' and that it really is not a fit subject for conversation. That kind of thinking would provoke a lot of hearty laughter from the people of Vilcamba, Ecuador or the people of Transcaucasia who enjoy sex continuously to the end of their lives (at around 125) and have babies in their 90's.

Someone has the wrong slant on sex and it certainly isn't the gracefully aging people in the various Shangri-las around the world. They know that sex is the most natural thing in the world (not to mention the most delightful, as well) and they heartily enjoy it. They are also aware that it keeps them young and prolongs their life span. Which is a welcome side effect.

One of the problems, here in America, is that we are all still suffering the effects of our Puritan heritage. Several hundred years of flinching at the term 'sex' has left its mark.

MASTURBATION

So much guilt has been implanted that most people are ashamed to admit that they have sexual fantasies. If they were questioned about it, they would vehemently deny that they ever indulged in such a 'degrading' activity. Just as most people deny that they masturbate, when the fact is that most people do both and do them quite frequently. They also suffer with guilt for not being able to "break the insidious habit'.

They might as well try to break the insidious habit of breathing. The plain fact is that sexual desire, sexual fantasy and masturbation are normal and enjoyable aspects of living, just as intercourse is. We are all sexual beings, awake or asleep. It's natural for us to be sexually involved almost from the moment we're born until the day we die. To deny this is to deny a major portion of our lives.

130

There is a sexual tonality to almost every activity we engage in—as infants, as children, as adolescents, as adults, as middle-aged people and as older people. It's always there. It does no good to deny it—*and it does a lot of harm when we try*.

Sexuality is a totality of being in which actual sexual intercourse only plays a part. You can have considerable sexual activity without actual copulation. Sex does not mean one particular act. It does not mean that a man has to place his erect penis in a woman's receptive vagina and then thrust it back and forth until he or she or both of them in concert, achieve a climax. To think this is to deny the entire range of pleasurable sexual activity that can take place without actual sexual intercourse.

THE ORGASM

Incidentally, the climax, as great as it is, is a *climax*. So many people seem to engage in sex with a frantic urge to achieve climax as soon as possible. That makes as much sense as rushing to a concert in time to hear the thundering climax of a symphony and leaving the hall perfectly satisfied. Sexual activity is not synonymous with orgasm. Orgasm should be considered the superb dessert that tops a magnificent feast. Your orgasm is not the feast.

Yet that's all we seem to hear these days.

Sexuality is also sensuality, a profound delight in touching, kissing, caressing, tasting and inhaling the aroma of your partner in sex. Sexuality is a profound expression of erotic communion, of joining with, of melting into a loved one and, together, creating a time out of time that reaches into the depth and breadth of being.

There's a lot more to sex than a healthy orgasm. It's a lot more than swift climaxing. Most people have no idea of the enormous range of delight that sex offers. Just as most people have no idea of how to masturbate. They simply rape themselves.

That's not surprising since they carry over the same idea of climax. Most masturbation is done quickly, furtively and with a completion compounded of relief and disgust. That's really a piece of sheer insanity when you stop to think about it. Most men seem to flog their penis as though it was an insensible piece of meat that must be forced to ejaculate immediately.

Most women treat their clitoris just as badly. None of these *self-rapists* have the slightest idea of the satisfaction that can be derived by a subtle approach to masturbation. Just as they have no idea of the satisfaction that can be achieved by approaching intercourse with consideration and finesse.

Just as people everywhere deserve the government they have, so people who use a brutal approach to sex deserve exactly what they get from sexual congress.

Sex, some wit remarked, is 99% psychological and 1% physiological. It happens to be true. Most of sex is in your head. If your head isn't on right—neither is your sex. Most men are impotent because they have an improper attitude towards sex. They consider sex as a 'performance' rather than an engagement. Their idea of 'performing' is to achieve an enormous erection at will; then to skewer a helpless female with it, engage in violent motion and ejaculate just as violently.

IMPOTENCE AND FRIGIDITY

Such men, who equate their virility with the hardness of their penis are born victims of early impotency. Such men can be rendered impotent swiftly by any discerning and angry woman. Once the seed of doubt as to their virility has been planted such men are condemned to continuous impotency.

Considerable psychotherapy is the only thing that will help them to achieve erection. Yet this is the one area that they will avoid because they cannot bear the thought of seeking psychiatric help. They're convinced that it's a physical disability.

So called 'frigidity' in women is another matter entirely. In most women it's simply that their husbands are not able to arouse them sexually. This does not mean they cannot be aroused by another man. They can (and are) frequently aroused by strangers, neighbors, relatives. Most women (thanks to sex taboos implanted by parents) are unable to seek and find sexual gratification without enormous guilt.

Some are able to enjoy these extramarital relationships and, because of them, are able to maintain their marriage. Others, once having tasted the joys of natural sex, leave their partners and seek another—or just *leave*—period.

Some women simply do not enjoy sex with a man. They prefer sex with another woman. This sort of an alliance is much easier to achieve because the world does not look askance at two women who spend an afternoon or an evening together.

Most women, in marriage, 'fake' ecstacy for the benefit of their husband's ego. It also makes the marriage more bearable if their husband is happy and contented. However, this kind of marriage is a sham and sooner or later it will come apart at the seams. Honesty—in sex—as in life, is the best policy.

The next question is—*why do women marry men that do not arouse them sexually?* The fact is that most women are aroused in the beginning—not by the man they married—but by sex itself. In their innocence they equate sex with their husbands and only find out when it's too late that they've made a mistake. So, instead of splitting up, then and there, they decide, out of misplaced pride, to 'make the best of it'—but they rarely do. They just manage to postpone the inevitable.

The idea of living to 100 or longer in that kind of situation is unthinkable to most women. Also to most men who had the reverse of the situation.

I would simply suggest that there is no reason why you should continue to live in an intolerable situation regardless of whether you are going to live to be 100. Why not now?

ENJOY LIFE NOW

Regardless of your age, now is the best time of your life. Enjoy it. I don't care if you're 90 right now, there is life and loving to be enjoyed. Sex is not a memory, as you are well aware. You still have sexual fantasies, you still have a sexual desire and you are still capable of achieving an entirely satisfactory sexual relationship. You see, the myth of the diminished desire as you get older has been destroyed forever, You can come out of the closet now. The artificial veil of silence and shame no longer exists. Start enjoying your life the way you were meant to enjoy it.

Only a very few things stand in your way. One is sexual health. That can be improved tremendously through proper diet. Just as your physical health needs a balanced diet with proper nutrition and vitamins—so does your sexual health. Obviously, if you enjoy excellent health, your sex health will also be in excellent condition. However, there are certain vitamins that can help you to regain sexual vigor.

Since your liver plays a key role in maintaining the proper estrogen-androgen balance (male/female hormone balance) then you should be careful to get vitamin A—you can do that mostly with sunlight—or small, occasional doses of cod liver oil. Remember that vitamin A is stored in the body so beware of overdosage.

If you lack vitamin B you can suffer degeneration of sexual glands. Check the vitamin pages in Chapter Five for the best sources of vitamin B and eat your way back to sexual health.

Vitamin E is another important vitamin for sexual vigor.

Since sexual excitement causes considerable excretion of calcium, you should look into a proper food source when you begin to engage in sexual intercourse with some regularity.

APHRODISIACS

Believe me, there are no such things as aphrodisiacs.

A healthy body and a healthy mind will provide all the stimulant you could possibly want.

You may read about things like cantherides (Spanish Fly) and Yohimbine which is made of the bark of a South African tree, as being 'true' aphrodisiacs. They are not. These substances cause intense inflamation of the gastro-urinary tract and rather than turning a man or a woman into a person with an insatiable craving for sex, *it can cripple or kill them.* So forget about any of these so called aphrodisiacs.

Remember, each new way you discover to increase and enhance your sexuality and your sexual pleasure will also increase your life expectancy. Think about that the next time you hear someone say that sex is strictly for the very young.

KEEP AN OPEN MIND

There are a thousand delights you have not discovered as yet. Did you know that the entire human body is an erogenous zone? It is. There is hardly a part of your body that will not respond to an intimate caress. Try it and see. Then try it on your sex partner. Try a gentle and prolonged approach to the genital area and watch your partner's excitement rise in direct ratio to the time you take to reach the genitals. Start your caresses at the toes and work up slowly and tantalizingly.

Don't limit your lovemaking to the bedroom. It's more exciting when it begins in another part of the house or apartment. An unexpected caress can also be exciting.

Start to think about yourself in terms of sex. Here are some things to think about. *Don't just read them.* Take a notepad and doodle some thoughts while you're thinking.

INTIMACY

Are you able to give and receive intimacy? Have you ever really allowed another person to know all about you? Are you secure enough to just be yourself and admit who and what you are to another person? Can you accept the same honesty from that other person?

Do you realize that if you cannot do either, then you will never truly accept yourself or accept anyone else? Until you learn to love, admire and respect yourself, you cannot expect anyone else to, nor can you truly love, admire and respect anyone else. Until you are ready to enter a relationship with all your defenses down you cannot begin to experience the full ecstacy and joy of sexual relationships. Sure it takes a lot of courage to lay yourself bare and defenseless—but the rewards are worth your courage. *Do you dare to be youself?*

NEED

Have you ever thought about *your own sexual needs?* Do you enter a sexual relationship with the idea of giving only rather than receiving? Can you accept the gift of orgams without feeling compelled to give an orgasm in return? Do you feel guilty if your lover brings you to a climax at times and then permits you to fall asleep without any demands at all that you return the compliment? Do you believe that you have equal rights when it comes to needs and wants?

SEXUAL GENDER

Do you accept your sexual gender? Do you look for ways to enhance your gender? Do you deliberately try to be more sexually desirable? *Are you comfortable in being what you are?* Would you like to change? Would you like your partner to change? Could your partner's sexuality be enhanced? Are you comfortable with your partner? Do you enjoy sex with your partner all the time or only at certain times?

NAKED PLEASURE

Do you enjoy being naked? Have you ever looked at yourself in the mirror when you are naked? Does the sight please you? Do you enjoy seeing your partner naked? Does it excite you? Have you ever thought about looking at erotic pictures while you and your partner are naked? Would you enjoy having a picture of your naked partner? Would you like your partner to have a naked picture of you? Does thinking about being naked excite you? Have you ever fantasized about being naked?

ORGASM

Is having an orgasm important to you? Have you ever engaged in intercourse and enjoyed it thoroughly without reaching orgasm? Have you ever achieved satisfactory orgasm through masturbation? Do you enjoy your orgasm? Do you enjoy bringing your sex partner to orgasm? Do you 'let yourself go' during orgasm? Do you ever reach a point during intercourse where you just want the lovemaking to go on and on and never reach orgasm? Do you know how you reach orgasm? *Do you know why you don't have an orgasm?*

MASTURBATION

Do you enjoy masturbating? Do you feel guilty afterwards? How many different ways can you masturbate? Where do you enjoy masturbation the most? Do you ever watch yourself while you masturbate? *Do you masturbate slowly and lovingly· or do you just rape yourself and get it over with?* Do you enjoy being masturbated by your sex partner? Do you enjoy masturbating your sex partner? Do you ever have fantasies about masturbating? Would you enjoy watching your partner masturbate? Would you enjoy having your partner watch you?

TOUCHING

Do you enjoy being touched? Do you enjoy touching? Do you like to communicate your feeling to others by touching? Do you enjoy touching your lover? Do you enjoy it when your lover touches you? Are you excited by touching? Are there certain areas that excite you more than others? Does your lover know where these areas are? Do you know where your partner's excitement areas are? Do you enjoy touching yourself? Can you turn yourself on by touching yourself?

VARIETY

Do you always have sex the same way? Or do you try new and varied ways to make love? When was the last time you made love at a drive-in movie? At the beach in the sand? In the bathroom? In a pool at night? When was the last time you went swimming in the nude? How many different ways have you tried? Are you willing to experiment with new ways?

SEXUAL DIALOGUE

Do you ever talk to your partner about sex? Do you enjoy discussing sexual fantasies with your partner? Do you talk at all while you are having intercourse? Do you ever guide your partner during sex? Do you ever request certain delights? Ever ask your partner to request certain delights? Do you ever let go and verbalize your delight in lovemaking? Do you ever tell your partner how you are feeling during intercourse? Does your partner ever tell you? How many different sounds do you make when you are having intercourse? Do you verbalize your orgasm? Do you talk about it afterwards?

You should have been doing a great deal of thinking after reading that material. Quite possibly your thinking will lead you to change because change is the essential ingredient to all growth. Growth leads to healthy new life and that, in turn, leads to a longer and more enjoyable life.

The changes you make need not be dramatic. They can be subtle and not readily noticeable at first but they can have impact on your sex life.

Here are some suggestions. I'm certain that once you put your mind to it you will come up with many more.

CHANGE THE WAY YOU DRESS

Wear different clothes than you usually wear. Give yourself a new and exciting look. You'll be amazed at the difference it will make in you—*and in your partner.*

CHANGE YOUR BODY STYLE

Try moving a little differently. Nothing dramatic, just a subtle change that can add excitement.

THINK OF NEW WAYS TO AROUSE

Stop treating your sex partner like an old hat. Try thinking of new ways to arouse your partner—at different times. Try to think of five erotic things you've never done before. Plan a surprise—there are any number of ways to surprise.

Change, as I said, is the key word. If you can change—you can grow and you learn to increase and expand your capacity for enjoyment you will find that life can be much more enjoyable and worth living. You will find increased pleasure in your sex life and in your social life. Your capacity for work and enjoying work will also increase. So start changing.

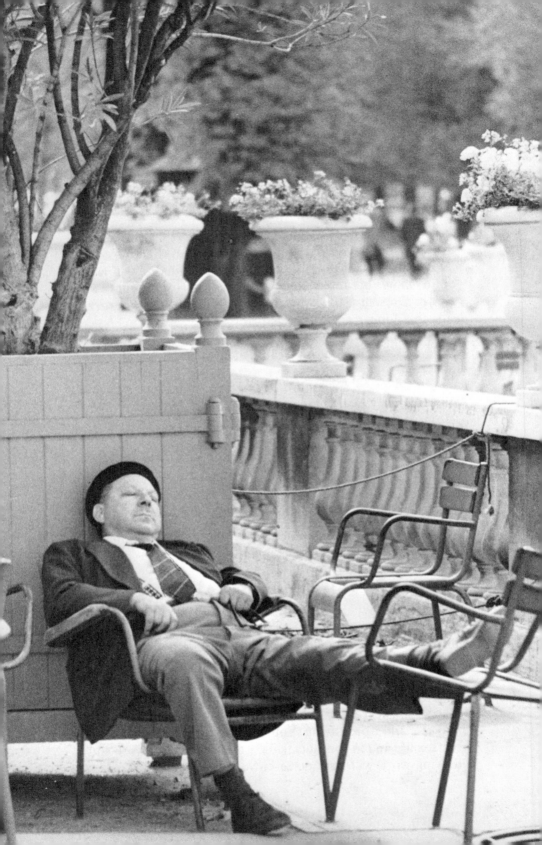

CHAPTER EIGHT

THE CHOICE OF STRESS OR SERENITY

He has not learned the lesson of life
who does not every day surmount a fear.
R.W. EMERSON

Stress is a peculiar word; it has many meanings. The unabridged edition of the Random House Dictionary offers 14 different definitions of the word 'stress' including these:

1. the physical pressure, pull or other force exerted by one thing or another; strain
2. the action on a body of any system of balanced forces, whereby strain or deformation results
3. any stimulus, as fear or pain, that disturbs or interferes with normal physiological equilibrium of an organism.

Although most people will, if asked, express the opinion that 'stress' is a bad thing, in reality *stress is a fundamental part of living*. Without stress there would be no life. What is generally meant by stress therefore is overstress, in which the victim is forced to pay a high price in terms of physiological and mental damage. So we will use the term in that sense throughout this chapter and thus avoid any misunderstanding.

The medical community now considers stress to be a national epidemic in American society. Most of the major causes of death (heart disease, stroke and cancer) have a direct link to the stress created by modern living. Yet, if stress is a natural state of life why does it cause damage to modern man?

The answer lies in the lack of use of the products of stress by modern man. One hundred thousand years ago, stress was part of man's survival kit. Sudden fear or anger triggered a 'stress condition and the body went on 'red alert' ready for 'fight or flight'. The heart begins pumping at 'full speed ahead' the blood vessels narrow considerably (to lessen the loss of blood in the encounter) and a package of adrenalin, blood sugar and cortisone is readied for use wherever the body needs it. If it's 'fight' the package goes to the arms and torso; if it's 'flight' the package goes to the legs.

That package, once delivered, could enable man to fight like a demon or run like a deer. Unfortunately modern man does neither. He just seethes with anger or gets sick with fear and the package settles into the stomach like a soggy lump and then he gets sick to his stomach. His blood pressure is sky high without any direct need or use, his respiration rate is way up and so is his pulse—in all—he's in a hyperstate but doesn't use any of this readiness.

If modern man could learn to use it—to run—jump up and down—to flail his arms—to engage in any strenuous physical activity, he would benefit tremendously. But he does nothing. He just stands there and burns and gets sick.

MODERN STRESS

Unlike our ancient ancestors who encountered widely spaced stress situations (and dealt with them in a healthy manner), modern man faces continuous stress from the time he wakes in the morning until he goes back to bed at night. The alarm clock jolts him awake; the kids scream and yell at breakfast; the garbage truck and the neighbor's car splits the morning air; the ride to the station is a nightmare; the subway ride is high decibels all the way; his office or factory is filled with the noise of telephones, loud speakers, machinery noise; and so it goes, from morning till night—noise, tension, stress situation after stress situation, with no end in sight.

When you add to the physical stress the continuous mental stress caused by the nature of work, the pressures of competition and the fear of losing a bonus, promotion or the job itself, it's little wonder that stress cuts down so many men and women in the prime of life. Nor is it any wonder that most Americans use some kind of tranquilizer such as alcohol, cigarettes, sleeping pills and tranquilizing drugs like valium, librium, miltown and the rest. Unfortunately, these 'tranquilizers' cause as much harm as the stress does and thereby compound the damage.

THE TYPE "A" PERSONALITY

Now, in addition to the stress caused by the environment and external stimulus, there is also the self-induced stress exhibited by individuals possessing what behavorial scientists call 'The Type A Personality.'

This particular personality is typified by the man or woman who believes that the only answer to pressure is to attempt to do everything now—today. This is the person that's filled with a continuous sense of urgency. In many respects this is a success-oriented person—who does manage to achieve considerable success but finds little time to enjoy it. Enjoyment and relaxing is put off to a future tomorrow—meanwhile, there's work to be done! It's hustle, hustle, hustle—make every moment count.

In test studies made recently the indication is that elimination of the type A personality would reduce the risk of heart disease by more than 31%. That's a considerable reduction. If we turn it around we see what a contribution type A stress makes in the high incidence of heart disease.

TRAUMAS

Now the environmental stress coupled with the type A stress is bad enough but there is more, much more to stress induction than that. There's also stress-triggered-response to early trauma (mental wounds) occasioned by frightening experiences that are only recognized by the subconscious mind—not the conscious mind. Here's a hypothetical example:

Suppose, as a very young child, we were terribly frightened by a tall man who chased us during a raging thunderstorm. The experience was so traumatic that we erased it from our conscious mind, *but it remains in our subconscious mind.* Just think of the number of stress-triggers that are cocked and ready to fire fear into us each time we encounter a facsimile of the original stimulus.

1. **Any tall man suddenly running toward us—even if he passes by us and is running after someone else—the fear is triggered.**
2. **A sudden, violent thunderstorm triggers fear—which you hide because you know that it's childish to be afraid.**
3. **Anyone suddenly running towards you.**

More and more people are beginning to understand that any unreasonable fear must have an original source. With luck and persistence, a psychiatrist or psychotherapist can uncover this original trauma and by inducing you to verbalize it, free you from the trigger-stimulus conditioning.

PHOBIAS

Take 'phobias' for example. There are about 62 different kinds of phobias ranging from acrophobia (fear of heights) to zoophobia (fear of animals) to do it alphabetically. Most psychiatrists are agreed that most phobias spring from an unpleasant (and forgotten) childhood experience. The phobia itself is developed as a defense against anxiety. The anxiety instead of being formless is displaced into something *concrete* and the anxiety is reduced somewhat. Although most people are fully aware of the unreasonableness of a phobia (fear) they are unable to control the sudden fear when faced with the object of the phobia. The sudden sight of an ordinary cat sends a shock of fear through a person suffering from ailurophobia. *Forcing a person to live with a phobia is not the answer.* Desensitization is. This works. It involves the use of suggestion, injections of tranqulizers while bringing the phobia object closer and closer—until finally the victim can be serene and tranquil while actually petting a cat—for example. Now while this may be comforting to know—the fact remains that phobias exist—that many people have them and thus suffer stress each time they encounter the phobia object. This can make life extremely difficult. There is the secondary stress factor of 'being afraid of being afraid' and then there is a closed circle of fear.

THE TWO BRAINS

Is there something that can be done? Something that we can do ourselves to overcome these various stress factors and become successful in our search for serenity? Yes, indeed.

We can begin by understanding that we have two different kinds of brains. That's right—two brains. The older brain in our skull is quite similar to the brain of an ordinary animal. It's very much like a computer that has been tuned and programmed to operate the various organs and glands of our body without any conscious effort on our part. In point of fact, many of the various processes that take place inside our body are completely beyond our conscious control.

Certain glands secrete certain substances on a continuous basis; the food and liquid we consume is changed into wide variety of substances; the bone marrow produces red blood cells—and on and on—without any direction at all from you or even awareness that these things are taking place.

This older brain, in addition to operating autonomously is also directly influenced by the thalamus (which has been called the seat of emotion). It is in this older brain that all the phobias, fears, anxieties and stress-triggers operate. All of the ancient instincts lie in this older brain. There is no logic or reason in this older brain just instinctive, emotionally toned reaction. It operates, for the most part, from previous conditioning—previous programming.

Our newer brain is quite different. It is able to reason, use logic, determine cause and effect, make judgements coolly and execute intricate tasks involving symbols—which are things created by the newer brain to 'stand for' other things.

Now although this newer brain cannot do very much (without extraordinary training) about the bodily functions, it can do a lot about the *emotional* activity of the older brain. It can, for example, either *reinforce* an emotional reaction or *override* the reaction and perform in spite of the misgivings and fears of the older, emotional brain.

143

FEAR

Fear is either real or imaginary; it is either logical and rational or illogical and irrational. Your older brain cannot distinguish between the two, it simply reacts, whereas your newer brain can see and apprecate the difference. This does not mean that an *untrained* newer brain can eliminate fear whether it's real or imaginary, because fear (and the physical reaction it triggers), is a *spontaneous* reflex. It happens whenever the older brain is presented with the fear-object (as in phobia-induced fear) or with the fear-situation.

For example, whenever a person afflicted with androphobia (fear of men) sees a man—any man—a stab of blind, unreasoning fear is induced immediately. Even though the newer brain can clearly see that the man is a friend or a relative who has always been kind and considerate, the older brain refuses to reduce the fear. The older brain cannot be reasoned with by an untrained newer brain. *It can be overriden by the newer brain.* In a way this is unfortunate because if the body responded to the fear and ran away from the fear-object, the body would be served in a healthy manner—meaning that all of the red-alert conditions in the body would be *employed* physically in a healthy way.

But the newer brain prevents this from happening and forces the body to function slowly or not at all *as though the situation were perfectly normal.* The situation is normal from a logical standpoint but not from the body's physical standpoint—and so damage is done. The heart is pumping blood madly but because there is little or no concurrent ingestion of oxygen (which would be the case in violent running) cells are deprived and die. The package of high-octane fuel that was assembled slowly disintegrates in the stomach (the worst place for it) and a sickening feeling is induced. The high blood pressure caused by the constricting of the blood vessels succeeds in producing a blinding headache.

LOGIC AND REASON

Logic and reason, which force the body to conform to the code of conduct imposed by modern society, are essentially the criminals responsible for murdering your body. That's the irony of modern living. We live in a world with the capacity for creating a thousand times the stress-situations faced by our ancient ancestors and yet, even though we could cope with it all, quite easily, on a primitive level, a code of behavior imposed by our newer brain prevents us from coping.

A dilemma, according to the dictionary, is a situation which requires a choice between two equally undesirable alternatives. Isn't that exactly what we have here? You're damned if you do and damned if you don't. If you react naturally and physically to a fear induced reflex you will, in short order be judged as a danger to civilized society and be incarcerated in some mental institution. On the other hand if you obey the customs and manners of society you will, in a relatively short period of time become a victim of stress and acquire one of the major stress-induced diseases which account for 67% of deaths.

THE ALPHA STATE

There is a way to solve this dilemma. There is a simple, effective way to cope with this terrible age of anxiety. It has nothing to do with drugs or tranquilizers. It will not harm or impair your body or brain. It will actually help to make your body healthier and permit your brain to function at increased capacity. It will most certainly extend your life span.

Best of all it costs you absolutely nothing. The most you will invest is a few hours of your time and the rewards will far exceed anything you could possibly imagine.

I'm talking about your innate ability to create a different state of mind called the ALPHA STATE of mind. Sometimes called the Alpha Dimension, this state of mind is the key to complete control of your older brain and through it, your entire body. *This isn't a state of mind that is unfamiliar to you because you enter the Alpha dimension at least twice a day from the time you're born until the day you die.* To understand it better, take a look at the following illustration:

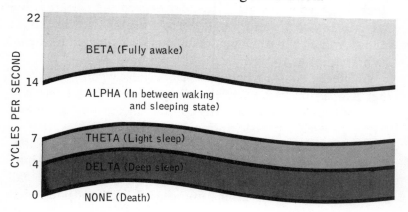

This illustrates the various brainwave frequencies which have been recorded on electroencephalograph (EEG) machines. BETA (from 22 to 14 cycles per second) is the normal frequencies produced by a human brain during the day when we are fully awake. When we go to sleep, the brainwave frequencies begin to diminish and when we reach the ALPHA state (between 14 and 7 cps) we are *approaching* sleep. We are not yet asleep. We begin to fall into a light sleep when the frequency of the brainwaves drop below 7 cps. This is the dreaming dimension where REM (rapid eye movements) disclose the fact that we are dreaming. When the brainwave frequencies fall below 4 cps we enter deep sleep. If the brainwaves cease entirely then we are clinically dead.

To return to the ALPHA state, it should be apparent that you pass through the Alpha dimension as you fall asleep each night and you rise up through it as you come awake.

Since this is a continuous state of affairs with every human it obviously is true for you. Therefore you are not unfamiliar with the Alpha dimension. In point of fact you have, unconsciously employed it on a number of occasions.

Here is a typical situation that must have occurred to you at some time in your life. Let's say that you heard the alarm, turned it off and instead of getting up immediately, decided to just lie there and enjoy the luxurious feeling of being neither awake or asleep. At the same time you said, something like this to yourself:

"This feels wonderful. But I'd better not keep lying here like this because I'll fall back to sleep and the next thing I know, I'll wake up and find that I have really overslept and I'll be late for work and I just can't afford to do that."

The next thing you know you bolt awake—look at the clock—and wow! It's late. You did oversleep and you are going to be late for work even though you rush around like mad to get ready. And all the while you're furious with yourself for being such an idiot as to oversleep.

You really couldn't help yourself because when you were in that Alpha dimension you actually gave yourself a *command* to oversleep. You were actually conducting auto-hypnosis and giving yourself a post-hypnotic suggestion.

Keep that in mind because we're going to return to it later. Right now we're going to show you how to enter the Alpha state deliberately instead of waiting until you begin to fall asleep at night. Why is this important? Well consider what happens when you are in an Alpha state. Your brainwave frequencies are much lower—about half the frequencies of the Beta state. This extra calm has a calming effect on your body. It actually *tranquilizes* the body. Can you imagine the benefits your body would receive it if could be plunged into a calm and tranquil state in a moment of crisis? *You will be able to do that when you become adept at creating the Alpha state at will.*

ALPHA STATE (Preparation)

In the beginning, you will have to create the proper environment that will induce relaxation. Later, when you become proficient at creating the Alpha state, you will induce relaxation through creation of the Alpha state in any environment. So follow these steps:

1. Find a place that is free of fear of interruption and is comfortable. If there is no such place then check into a motel. You must be completely secluded.
2. Your bodily comfort is extremely important. Little or no clothing is advisable. Loose pajamas or a night gown would be excellent. Remove your rings, watch, etc.
3. You may either lie down on the bed or floor or sit up in a comfortable chair with your feet propped up. Please use an open position, with your legs uncrossed and your hands loose and open.
4. Remind yourself, before beginning, that you have entered the Alpha dimension many times and will be able to do it again with ease.
5. Remind yourself that you have, in the past, given your subconscious mind (older brain) instructions and these instructions were followed to the letter.
6. Read the instructions on *how to exit from the Alpha state* before you begin your steps of entering the Alpha dimension.

ENTERING THE ALPHA STATE

If everything is ready; you are in a secure and secluded place; you are wearing little or no clothing, and you are lying or sitting in an open position, you can begin.

1. Close your eyes and begin to breathe deeply. Hold each breath for a count of 4 and then exhale slowly and, as you do, imagine that all the tension in your body is being expelled with each slow exhalation. Continue this type of breathing through all that follows.

2. After you have been breathing in this manner for awhile, start to visualize the number 5. Imagine that you have a piece of soft chalk and you are forming a large 5 on a large blackboard. Keep concentrating on seeing that big white 5 on the black background as you continue with your slow and deliberate breathing.
3. Once you can see the 5 fairly clearly, start saying mentally 'Five' each time you exhale. Do this 5 times.
4. Now begin to form a large white 4 on the blackboard. As soon as you can see it, start saying 'Four' mentally each time you exhale. Do this 4 times.
5. Now begin to write a large white 3 on the blackboard. As soon as you can see it, start saying 'Three' each time you exhale. Do this three times.
6. Now start forming the number 2 on the blackboard and when you can see it, start saying 'Two' each time you exhale. Do this three times.
7. Form the number 1, say 'One' three times.
8. You should, by now, be extremely relaxed. Silently remind yourself that you have entered the Alpha dimension and that you have entered into a state of calm that is healthy and healing. Tell yourself that you wish to remain in this state for a few minutes and that when you are ready you will leave this state. Remember that this particular state of mind is familiar to you because you have entered it many many times in the past. The only difference is that now you are controlling it. Now you are entering it because you *want* to rather than just having it happen to you.

In the beginning, as you become more familiar with and develop more ability to control the Alpha state, do not attempt anything more than simple suggestions to the older brain (the subconscious) and give your instructions just before leaving the Alpha state.

LEAVING THE ALPHA STATE

1. Now mentally tell yourself that you are preparing to leave the Alpha state. Tell yourself you will count slowly from 1 to 5 and that on the count of 5 you will open your eyes and feel wonderful; that you will be completely relaxed, free of all tension, healthier and contented.

2. Start to count slowly. 'One', 'Two', 'Three'—pause and remind yourself that you will open your eyes at the count of 5 and feel more relaxed and healthier than ever—then continue to 'Four' and then 'Five'.
3. Now, on the count of 5, with your eyes open, tell yourself *"I am wide awake, alert, free of tension, healthier and feeling better than I have in a long, long time."*

Now get up and walk around and taste the sensation of being in complete control, yet completely calm, with your mind clearer and more perceptive than it has ever been.

Make up your mind, at that point, that this is the way you want to live your life. Get dressed and go out for a walk, and while you're walking take note of how clear and sharp everything seems. Notice how keenly aware you are of colors you never noticed before. You are discovering what complete functioning is. You are beginning to discover how really wonderful life can be, if you learn to really live.

This is nothing new. The alpha state that you entered is one that has been known to Eastern culture for thousands of years. *This is what transcendental meditation is all about.* There are many doorways to the Alpha state. I've just shown you a simple way that's closest to the most natural way to enter the alpha dimension. Remember that you have been entering the alpha dimension all your life, without any training at all, each time you fall asleep or wake up.

Now, in addition to having it at your command any time you wish to enter it, you will begin to exercise power and control of your older brain and your entire body while in this unique state of mind.

Here are some of the things that you will be able to do anytime you feel the need or want:

ALPHA STATE BENEFITS

You can create:	You can enjoy:
Continuous peace of mind	Lower blood pressure
A sense of well being	Increased relaxation
Continuous energy	Absence of fatigue
A more tolerant attitude	Freedom from worry
An optomistic attitude	Freedom from tension

These, of course, are only a few of the things you will be able to do, once you achieve complete mastery of the Alpha state. Many people, once they become adept, are tempted to try to eliminate bad habits such as smoking and drinking.

A word of warning.

You can eliminate them quite easily but you will not solve anything by doing that. You must discover the *reasons* why you smoke or drink (or both) because if you merely eliminate the smoking or drinking you are merely eliminating the symptoms rather than the *cause.* I can assure you that you can easily eliminate both smoking and drinking through your Alpha state but may find yourself with something far worse.

First discover the cause. When you eliminate that you will find the need for smoking and drinking (or whatever you're into) will disappear.

Concentrate on becoming a calm, healthy, rational being through your Alpha state control and the rest will come forth by itself. Trust me. Remember the key words—moderation and regularity. Be moderate in your use of this new control and exercise it regularly. The ten benefits I've outlined can change your life for the better.

You must be aware that all *change* causes stress. It doesn't matter whether the change is good or bad—stress will occur. That's because living itself consists of change and involves stress. It's how you cope with stress that counts.

Here's an idea of how stress (good or bad situation-stress) is evaluated on a stress table based on a high of 100.

STRESS TABLE

EVENT SITUATION	IMPACT
Death of husband or wife	100
Divorce	73
Personal injury or illness (serious)	63
Marital separation	65
Jail term	63
Death of a family member	63
Marriage	55
Fired from job	50
Retirement	46
Pregnancy	45
Difficulty with sex	40
Conflict with in-laws	30
Change of residence	22
Change in finances	40

Death of a close friend	40
Business readjustment	40
Christmas	15
Change in sleeping habits	18
Change in recreation	20
Change in church activities	20
Change of personal habits*	25
Minor law violation	15
Begin or finish school	28

(*) Your new ways of eliminating or relieving stress will initially cause new stress.

HOW TO USE THE STRESS TABLE

At first glance, the stress table contents might just provoke a shrug and you might say, "That's interesting—but it's fairly obvious, isn't it? Some things cause more stress than others.

The point of the stress tables, particularly the fact that your attempt to change your life will also cause stress, *is that you cannot attempt to do too much at one time without getting way over your head.* Think a moment. Suppose you started adding up a number of different stress-situations—what would you have then? Trouble in a great big way. Let's start at the top. Take the death of a husband or wife—that's a big one—the biggest of all—right? But that stress-situation doesn't stop there—it could also entail a lot of *changes* such as a change of residence—change of finances—conflicts with in-laws—and on into the night. You see? If you add all of the stress situations together then you have a mighty big problem.

This is one of the reasons why most self-improvement programs fail so miserably. People try to change too much at one time. Each additional change brings more stress in addition to the basic stress caused by the attempt to change. *So don't try to change yourself and your stress situations overnight.* Take them one step at a time, comfortably and you'll be able to eventually eliminate all of them quite easily.

EMPLOYING THE ALPHA STATE

Using the Alpha state of the mind to control the older mind or subconscious is part of a branch of science that is thousands of years old. It has been used in magical and religious rites, in ancient and modern medicine and in modern day psychiatry. When used by someone else to control a person's subconscious mind it is called hypnosis. When used by a person to control his own subconscious mind it is called auto-hypnosis.

One of the most startling cases of the use of auto-hypnosis and hypnosis was a remarkable character named Count Alessandro di Cagliostro who suddenly appeared, almost, it seemed, out of nowhere and took the world by storm. He swept through Greece, Egypt, Arabia, Persia, Rhodes, Malta and Italy and apparently had the power to heal every known disease simply by looking or touching the afflicted person. His fame and wealth, by the time he reached Europe, was fabulous. He and his beautiful wife, traveled all over Europe during the middle of the 18th century and in spite of the extreme jealousy of the medical profession (because of his many successes) Cagliostro seemed invulnerable.

Then, unaccountably, he became embroiled in the diamond necklaces scandal which involved no less than the Queen of France, Marie Antoinette, and was arrested and thrown into the Bastille. Later, in Rome, he was condemned to death as a heretic, but that was commuted to life imprisonment.

The point is, Cagliostro was born the son of poor peasants in Palermo, Italy and yet, with no education became one of the most literate men of his time. He was fluent in virtually every known language, was a commanding, authoritative personage and apparently had the gift of healing. Where did he obtain this enormous power? Through hypnotism. He was apprenticed to an apothecary in a monastery and managed, in a short time, to acquire a considerable knowledge of chemistry, so it is quite likely that he also learned to read and write. He certainly learned about hypnotism and auto-hypnosis because he used it freely in all his travels. He also used his auto-hypnosis to learn new languages (which he was able to speak without any trace of accent whatever).

Oddly enough, at about the same time, there was an Austrian physician named Franz Anton Mesmer who developed a theory of animal magnetism (which was actually hypnotism) and devoted himself to curing diseases with this strange occult power he had.

Unfortunately, a commission of scientists and physicians appointed by the French governmetn denounced Mesmer as a fraud and ended his career abruptly.

Today, psychiatrists use hypnosis, either induced by oral

means or by the injection of so-called 'truth serums' like sodium amytal, which permit direct access to the subconscious mind to uncover the mystery of the patient's hidden traumas.

Hypnosis has been employed in difficult childbirth or in cases where it was not possible to use drugs to induce an unconscious state for an operation.

The point is that there is nothing magical about using the Alpha state (or auto-hypnosis). It's a perfectly natural event and, when used with moderation and common sense, can be extremely helpful to achieving a harmonious relationship between your mental and physical condition.

ELIMINATING HEADACHES

Take the matter of headaches, which seem to be a modern day plague. Since most headaches (not all) are caused by tension you can remove the *physical* cause of the headache simply by placing yourself in an Alpha state. Once in that state you can calmly assess the reason for the headache. It might be the prospect of an unpleasant task—the visit of someone you don't like—the impending examination at school. It could be any number of reasons, but once you discover exactly what it is, it will cease to bother you. Placing yourself in an Alpha state immediately to relieve the headache is wise because it is difficult to think clearly with a pounding headache. Once you are in a calm state it is quite simple to analyze the reason for the headache and eliminate it.

MIND AND BODY

Once again, it becomes clear that we are *one single unit* with physical, psychological and spiritual dimensions. Each area contributes to the total harmony of the person. When we are physically fine, but mentally distressed, we can feel completely exhausted. On the other hand, poor physical health can threaten mental balance.

When the mind and body are kept in harmonious rhythm, our chances for happy longevity are greatly enhanced.

It is important in the practice of self-regulation to *learn passive awareness.* The alpha level cannot be willed or forced.

Don't try to analyze, as this will block alpha and keep you in the actively aware Beta level.

Don't try to hurry your progress. Proceed slowly and comfortably to achieve efective results.

Become aware of your natural body rhythms. Note the times of day in which you feel quiet; the times you feel brimming with energy. You can also find a pattern in your mental alertness and dullness. Keep a written record, and you will have a wonderful tool to help you toward self-regulation.

Each step we take leads to a harmonious equilibrium. We experience a total rest of the body unit.

When practicing self-regulation, an erect spinal column prevents sleepiness and aligns body energies. (Soon you will be able to do it anywhere.)

A simple sitting posture in a chair (which provides spinal support) seems best for most people. Hands may rest quietly on the arms of the chair, or, palms down on thighs.

If your body is limber from faithful exercise, you may choose a *yoga-like sitting posture without spinal support.*

Other people *sit on the floor with legs stretched out.*

It is important to *avoid a sleep-inducing position.* (Otherwise you may very well fall asleep.)

Be sure (especially during initial training) to seek out a place where you are free from harrassment of any kind. It should be quiet and secluded. Room temperature should be comfortably warm. Lighting should be moderate—neither too harsh nor too dark. All drafts should be eliminated.

In the beginning, the person learning self-regulation will find it helpful to use the same familiar place each time he or she seeks alpha-relaxed-consciousness. Just as certain environmental cues now cause tension, environmental cues can also be paired in association with pleasure as well. If you return to a spot where you have fond memories—you will more than likely feel good. The importance of practice in the same place at the start can not be stressed enough.

After the Alpha state becomes a fixed part of your daily routine, you will be able to achieve it anywhere . . . even a noisy and crowded waiting room or train station.

The following profile can be taken once a month to show individual progress. Use only for *self-encouragement,* not as a test on which you try for "good marks". Remember. *Progress,* is important not perfection!

MIND/BODY CONTROL PROFILE

1. Am I able to relax?
2. Do I become unaware of body feelings?

3. Did my mind wander?
4. Did my surroundings intrude?
5. Was I always *passively* aware?
6. Did I remain awake?
7. Did I experience deep comfort?

ADD SCORE IN THE FOLLOWING MANNER: 1=sometimes, 3=frequently, 4=always. When you have progressed *slowly* forward to a score of 35 or more, you will know you are getting great results!

The natural gifts you can expect as you progress are many. You will enjoy a noticeably different attitude and a wellspring of energy. You will be freed intellectually and spiritually to form more creative ideas.

You may enjoy physical proof of some of the bodily gifts you acquire through self-regulation. The following test is fun to try after your score on the MIND/BODY CONTROL PROFILE has reached 20 or more. You can of course try it at any time.

CONTROL YOUR PULSE

Lower your pulse rate in the following way. Before you do this exercise, take a reading of your pulse (as shown earlier in the book). Record it.

Following the instructions given, enter the alpha state of relaxed consciousness. You are then ready.

Concentrate on the blood flowing through your veins. As you relax, think about *slowing down circulation.* Concentrate on your heartbeat. Try to control it ever so slightly. Focus on blood circulation again. *Slowly. Slowly.* Think about all the different activities within your body beginning to slow down. Focus on resting completely.

Tell yourself that when you return to Beta level, you will have a lower pulse rate. Slowly leave alpha state. Measure your pulse and compare. See. You *are* in control! Here is another test to help you see the reality of your mind-over-body control.

BREATHING CONTROL

Everyone associates slower breathing with relaxation, and you can easily regulate your breathing and lower the respiration rate. Record your breaths per minute.

Enter the alpha state as instructed.

Become aware of the sound and feel of your breathing. Concentrate on relaxing your lungs and . . . letting go. Think of slowing down your breathing. Slow down more. Gradually inhale and exhale less. (Your state of complete passive awareness requires less oxygen.)

Tell yourself that your respiration rate will remain lowered for a bit after you return to active awareness. Slowly bring yourself out of the alpha state.

Record your breaths per second and compare!

The evidence you have found should help you in your potential for more and more "imaginary" experiences. You are increasing your inner sensory awareness.

As your ability to enter the Alpha dimension strengthens and as you begin to gain more and more control of your older brain and, through it, your body itself, you will begin to realize that there is literally nothing that you cannot do with your body.

A word of caution.

Pain is an important symptom. It's a signal that something is wrong. *Do not simply eliminate the pain and forget about it.* That's the most dangerous thing you can do. A friend of mine, who was quite adept in Alpha state manipulation of the body, developed a severe toothache in the middle of a conference. He excused himself, left the room, put himself into an Alpha state, removed the pain from his jaw and returned to the very important conference. In the days that followed, because of the intense nature of the work he was involved in, *he completely forgot about the pain that he had removed.*

When he finally went to the dentist he was in real trouble. The infection had eaten into the jawbone to a considerable depth. If it had gone much further there is every reason to believe that as he bit down, the jawbone would have snapped.

He was lucky. You may not be. Do not remove pain and then forget about it. Find out why the pain is there. If you must remove it for emergency purposes then remove it *for a specified period of time*. That way, it will come back and remind you if you forget.

Many physicians are now turning to the use of meditation— which is the Alpha state—to relieve, reduce and in some cases, eliminate allergic reactions. This is understandable because, as we pointed out earlier, many allergies are really phobias.

Psychosomatic illness, which, in a way, also resemble phobias since they have no physical cause, can also be eliminated with Alpha state action and auto-suggestion.

The language you use when you address your older brain must be simple, direct and concrete. Do not be vague or wordy. If you feel hesitant or at a loss for words then write down everything that you want to say. Then rewrite it several times. Each time you rewrite it try to eliminate unnecessary words. The best way is to pretend that you are sending a telegram and that each word costs one dollar. Make your commands in short declarative sentences. Don't use "I"—use the personal pronoun "YOU" as for example:

"You will wake up on the count of five. You will be fully awake, fully refreshed and fully alert. One. Two. Three. Remember, on the count of five you will be awake and your eyes will open. Four. You will be awake and fully refreshed, fully alert. Five. Open your eyes. You are fully awake and fully refreshed, and fully alert. Enjoy it."

Be direct, positive and fully confident that you will be obeyed. If you do, you will have no trouble at all with your older brain. It's used to being commanded. Whether you realize it or not you have been commanding it all of your life.

Whenever you have thought (thoughts are commands to the older brain) that it would be nice if you could stay home for awhile instead of going to work, your older brain assumes that is a direct command and obliges you. It can give you a range of excuses for staying home from a bad chest cold, to the flu, or possibly a badly sprained ankle. **YOUR OLDER BRAIN WILL DELIVER JUST ABOUT ANYTHING YOU WANT IT TO—SO BE CAREFUL IN YOUR REQUESTS.**

Most people, who have never had any knowledge of the power of the older brain in delivering exactly what has been asked, are really puzzled at the odd things that happen to them. They cannot understand how they suddenly become almost dangerously clumsy.

How many times have you heard someone say—"I knew that would happen if I did so and so?" *Are you getting the picture now?*

REPETITION

There is an advertising maxim that says: Repetition is reputation. As simplistic as that sounds, it happens to be perfectly true. If something is repeated enough, people tend to believe it. "Twonkies are GOOD for you." Keep that up long enough and after awhile people will say, "Everybody KNOWS that Twonkies are good for you." Right?

So each repetition of your auto-suggestion session will help to reinforce your control. Naturally, one of the best times to do it is just before you fall asleep at night and just before you wake up in the morning. In each instance you pass through the Alpha state naturally. So use each one of these naturally induced states to reinforce a particular auto-suggestion. You'll be amazed at how it begins to work.

ON BEING CHEERFUL

Let's take the matter of being cheerful and pleasant. The odd part is that when you are cheerful and pleasant you begin to affect everyone around you. They tend to become much more pleasant and don't really know why. So if you begin to work on becoming a cheerful, pleasant person, you will begin to affect all of the environments in which you live and work or play.

You will find, as you begin to gain more control over yourself that you are also beginning to gain more control over your different environments. As you change, they will change. Then, instead of dreading the thought of going to work you will look forward to it. Instead of dreading the thought of coming home you will look forward to it. The world will become an entirely different place when you start to enjoy it every day. Stress situations will begin to disappear because you will begin to eliminate them.

As the stress situations disappear your life expectancy will begin to rise and so will your health and happiness. It really is that simple. You'll see as you become better and better at inducing your Alpha state and your auto-suggestion control.

Remember when we spoke of the importance of language and *what we tell ourselves.* When you run into the myriad little hurdles and disappointments of life, try saying this to yourself: "IT REALLY DOESN'T MATTER".

This approach may seem simplistic and even silly. But I will guarantee that a faithful use of this simple tool will change your mind after only a few weeks. Simple or not, *it works!*

Try some other verbal instructions. In the morning, as you dress for the day, *program yourself positively.* Say:

1. **"Today I will definitely be more relaxed than yesterday."**
2. **"I have good control over my emotions."**
3. **"I feel immune to worry today."**
4. **"I am calm and composed today."**

Each individual will come to know the specific types of input they require. Are you often forgetful? Tell yourself that you will be efficient and remember all necessary things. Keep all suggestions positive and simple. Try only one or two statements at one time and focus momentarily on *believing* them. They can quickly become self-fulfilling prophecies... and you the beneficiary of a life-long inheritance of strength.

While on the subject of language, I would like to suggest a regular inventory or housekeeping, to clear out all the bad or negative messages we give ourselves that unfortunately can also become self-fulfilling. Do you ever say to yourself...

1. *"With my bad luck, such and such will happen."*
2. *"I get all the bad breaks."*
3. *"I just can't bear it another minute."*
4. *"I can't seem to cope."*
5. *"I woke up on the wrong side of the bed today."*
6. *"I'm no good for anything when I get up in the morning."*
7. *"Gee... I could* never *(ride a bike, drive a car, etc.)*
8. *"I'll never make it to be a hundred years old."*

Be your own best friend. *Encourage* yourself even when the going gets rough. Like the little train engine in the children's book who chugged up the mountain saying "I think I can... I think I can" you will find to your delight that mountains are rarely as high as they seem at first... and no problem at all for a winner like you!

TO SLEEP OR NOT TO SLEEP

That's the question that troubles a considerable number of Americans if we consider how many millions of sleeping pills are sold in these United States each year. If you are one of the sleepless horde and are taking any one of the 'over the counter' sleeping aides, you're wasting your money.

If these 'sleeping aides' had enough active substance in them to put you to sleep they couldn't be sold as non-prescription drugs. Ergo, they don't, therefore they're a fraud and you're being ripped off when you buy them—so save your money.

You're right when you worry about not sleeping. Sleep is a necessity, not a luxury. The question is: How much sleep do you really need? There is no such thing as a standard number of hours of sleep. Every human being is different not just in physical characteristics, but mentally, as well. There are no two lives exactly alike, no two environments exactly alike. You may feel that because you don't get eight hours sleep that you're depriving your body of the rest it needs. That's utter nonsense. Too much sleep can be as harmful as too little. I've had people come to me and say, *"I had ten hours sleep last night and I'm still tired."*

Why not? Most of that ten hours was spent in continuous twisting in turning as the body kept trying to avoid the inevitable consequences of a static position. Why do you suppose doctors try to get their patients on their feet so soon.

Stop fretting about being unable to sleep and take advantage of it. Catch up on the reading you keep wanting to do but never have the time. Study something you always wanted to study. If that doesn't please you, then practice your Alpha state. You can get more rest with ten minutes of complete relaxation than you can in ten hours of crawling around your bed.

You can forget about the "need to repair the body" routine. If your body waited until you went to sleep to repair itself you'd be dead in a year. The body repairs itself continuously.

The only reason you really have to sleep is to *dream*. There is hard evidence to show that persons who are prevented from dreaming will, in a relatively short time, become psychotic. So 'dreams' are the most important factor in sleep—not rest. You can rest anytime you want to. Many people get by with ten minute naps here and there and, at the most, two hours of actual sleeping time. They use the extra time to procure all sorts of work that the ordinary 'sleep trapped' person hasn't got the time for. Think about that, the next time you're worrying yourself to death because you can't get to sleep.

HOW MUCH SLEEP?

Think about this, too: If a person gets eight hours of sleep each night of his life then, at the age of 90, that person will have spent 30 years unconscious. *Thirty years!* Can you imagine what you could do with 30 years of spare time?

The fact of the matter is that most people sleep to escape life. That's right—sleep is an excuse for the majority of people. It gives them an excuse not to think about how bloody bored they are with life. It's a chance to stop worrying about all the idiotic things they worry about. A chance to shut out the nagging wife or the whining husband; to be free of the screaming, howling monsters that pass for children in our society. I don't blame them, I just want them to realize what they're doing.

I just want them to stop and think: If the life I'm living is so bad that I have to blot it out—why don't I just get out and find a better kind of life?

People who persist in staying in an intolerable situation remind me of the good old Southern boy who had a dog that howled all the time. When I asked him why the dog howled he said, "'*Cause he's just plain lazy.*"

"Lazy? Why would his being lazy make him howl?"

"'*Cause,*" the good old boy said with a sly grin, "'*cause he's asettin' on a thorn and he's too lazy to move.*"

There's an awful lot of people settin' on a thorny marriage and are just to lazy to move—so they howl and sleep. Think about that a little. It will get to you after awhile.

Now, if you're the one person in ten thousand who doesn't have a situational cause for insomnia, then here are some tips for sleeping whenever you want to sleep.

SLEEP TIPS

1. Drink slightly warmed milk. That's not an old wives' remedy it's a scientific fact. Recent analysis of milk has revealed certain substances which induce sleep.
2. After you drink the slightly warmed milk, read a dull book. There's nothing like a dull book to put you to sleep.
3. Read the dull book in bed (if possible). If not, because your dragon of a mate will scream to high heaven about

the bloody light, then read it on the couch in the living room. Be sure to put a blanket over you because your body temperature drops like a stone when you sleep and you could get a chill.

4. Never fight for sleep or try to force yourself to sleep, that's a sure fire way to stay awake.

5. Don't smoke while you're reading because you'll set yourself and the house on fire. Besides the cigarette smoke will interfere with your sleep inducement.

6. When you decide that you're ready, turn out the light and relax. Take long, deep breaths and think about the laziest scene you can imagine. Try to picture a long, white beach without a soul on it. You're lying in the hot sand, staring at the monotonous washing of the beach by slow, indolent waves. I imagine you'll be able to count about seven waves before you fall asleep.

ALPHA STATE SLEEP

This is a cinch and it will give you good practice with your Alpha state conditioning. Just get into position—on your back, relaxed and open and start your deep breathing exercises. Now start to form your number 1. with chalk on the blackboaad. As you begin your countdown at the word 'sleep' in this manner: One-sleep, Two-sleep. Three-sleep. I can guarantee that you won't get past chalk number 4 before you're fast asleep. Incidentally, the reason you *reverse* the countdown when you're using the Alpha state for sleep inducement is to prevent conditioning. Otherwise, every time you use the Alpha state to use auto-suggestion, you'll fall asleep before you can give yourself the commands.

Once you get the hang of Alpha state sleep you can forget your expensive sleeping aides or sleeping pills, because you'll never need them again.

Just remember, the proper use of your Alpha state conditioning can be your best defense against every stress situation in your home, your business and your social life. That conditioning, plus regular exercises and a proper diet can only prolong your life span, but it can help you to enjoy the added years which, in the long run is what you really want out of life.

In our next chapter we're going to discuss some of the ways that Astrology can help you to understand yourself better and through this understanding, avoid some of the pitfalls and hurdles that may rob you of the extra years you deserve.

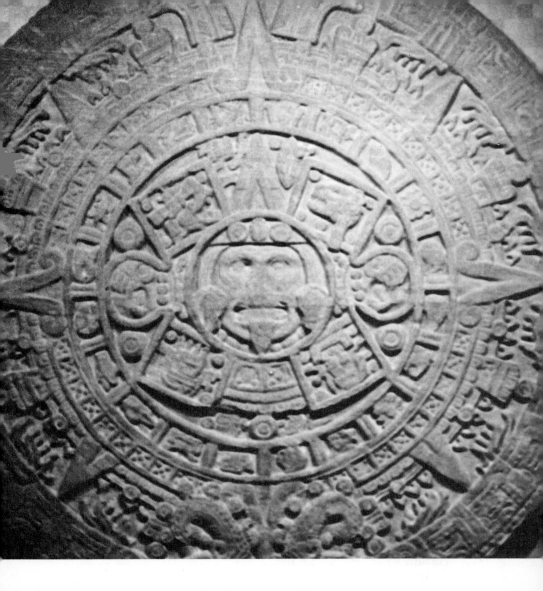

CHAPTER NINE

USING ASTROLOGY
TO LIVE LONGER

*Astra regunt homines, sed
regit astra Deus.*
(The stars rule men but God rules the stars.)
Medieval Proverb

Astrology has played a part in the development of mankind almost from the beginning of literacy. The pendulum of popular opinion with regard to astrology seems, in recent years to be swinging towards greater acceptance. Be that as it may I am not going to try to pursuade you that it is, or is not, a science. I am not going to throw out the baby with the bathwater, either.

There are certain aspects about astrology that can be helpful to you in your quest to lengthen your life span. Regardless of the truth or falsehood of astrology, per se, there is strong and continuous evidence that some aspects of it have validity.

Take the matter of the 'early warning system' with regard to certain physical weaknesses that astrology provides. Let us suppose, for the moment, that it is true that each person born under a particular sign of the zodiac has a predisposition to certain physical weak spots in his body. If this is true, then it would be helpful to know about those weak areas and take care to avoid disease or weakness where they are concerned.

Let us suppose that this aspect of astrology is *not* true. Would there be any benefit in taking precautions against weakness in those areas? Of course. All preventive measures are useful.

So let's assume that astrology is right about this 'early warning system' and use that information to our advantage. In the same manner, we might also take advantage of the general information astrology offers with regard to our basic personalities. Naturally this information is general because your sun sign is only a small part of your overall personality influence. However, the general indications are fairly accurate in many cases and, again, it can't hurt you to guard agains certain weaknesses, can it?

Many doctors have become willing to include astrology as an added *diagnostic aid*. And, while this may seem puzzling, anything that can prove helpful in the successful identification of illness should be meat for the open-minded to chew.

This is not to say that the reader should ever rely upon self-diagnosis of any kind. Professional medical checkups, as previously discussed, are a *must* for any intelligent program designed to promote longevity.

But the ancients may have known some truths that have been hidden from light with the passage of time. It is interesting to consider how the stars may influence our comfort and health.

Did you know, for example that recent resarch in New York revealed the fact that there is a definite correlation between disturbances in the earth's magnetic field and an increase in mental illness? Growing evidence leads us to believe that the sun and moon have a direct influence on our blood.

In some circles, astrology has become an accepted adjunct to psychiatry and psychology. Famed scientist, Dr. Carl Jung once noted *"Astrology is assured of recognition from psychology without further restrictions because it represents the summation of all psychological knowledge of antiquity."*

Somebody out there thinks there's something to it. So let's keep an open mind and look into this business of the possibility that there is a relationship between your sun sign and your physical and mental health.

If, for some reason, you have no idea of your astrological sun sign, here is a table for your convenience. Even though it's hard for me to believe, at this late date, that there is any man, woman or child alive who doesn't know his or her particular sign of the zodiac.

NAME	SYMBOL	DATES
ARIES	RAM	Mar 21 thru April 19
TAURUS	BULL	April 20 thru May 20
GEMINI	TWINS	May 21 thru June 21
CANCER	CRAB	June 22 thru July 21
LEO	LION	July 22 thru Aug 21
VIRGO	VIRGIN	Aug 22 thru Sept 22
LIBRA	SCALES	Sept 23 thru Oct 22
SCORPIO	SCORPION	Oct 23 thru Nov 21
SAGITTARIUS	ARCHER	Nov 22 thru Dec 21
CAPRICORN	GOAT	Dec 22 thru Jan 20
AQUARIUS	WATER-BEARER	Jan 21 thru Feb 19
PISCES	FISH	Feb 20 thru Mar 20

There are your basic sun signs and as you may note, there is a span of time when these sun signs are in force. However, sometimes, when you are close to another sign, it might be a good idea to consider the physical weaknesses of the close sign as well as your own. In other words, spread your bet a little, it can't hurt.

Now we're going to do a brief run down on each sign. Please do not accept this material as being completely definitive. If you really want pinpoint information about yourself you will have to engage an astrologer to do a natal chart based upon the exact time of your birth and the exact latitude and longitude of your birth place. There are any number of astrologers who can do this—and there are computers that have been programmed to do it. So if that's what you want—go to it. Just so long as I have made it clear that I am not offering you that kind of deep assistance in the material that follows.

ARIES

This is one of the most exciting signs in the zodiac. Men and women born under this sign are dynamic personalities. They are extremely original—sometime too far ahead of their time. They blaze trails that others must follow because once they've shown the way they're off on another adventure. Their boundless energy can sometimes be their undoing because they are scornful of weakness in themselves and can push their bodies to the point of exhaustion. Although, because of their great strength of mind, they can carry on with illness and sick bodies that would fell an ox, in the end, if they are not careful, they too, can succumb. They are not immortal, although sometimes they think they are.

PHYSICAL ASPECTS:

There is a tendency to Headaches, Headcolds, Eye Strain, Dental Problems, Strokes, Fevers and Nervous Exhaustion.

All of the above can easily be avoided with self discipline, relaxation and a well-balanced diet. If the Arien person can practice moderation there is every reason to expect a long life span. However, it's difficult to convince Ariens of this.

TAURUS

This is one of the most stable signs. Taureans are strong, loyal, dependable and patient. They are the strength of the civilized world because they are the finest executives and the best employees. Here is your wise and conservative banker who understands the value of money and sound investment. Taureans are stable in domestic life and provide the world with marriages that last. On the negative side, Taureans like to eat and tend to overeat. They have excellent resistance to disease but once they become ill they take a long time to recover.

PHYSICAL ASPECTS

There is a tendency towards Colds and Throat Infections which should not be taken lightly since they may become chronic. The weak areas are the Neck, Ears and Sex Glands. Taureans can overcome many deficiencies through moderation in eating (avoiding fattening foods) and employing regular exercise.

GEMINI

This is a sign of the many-sided intellectual. Persons with this sign are extremely versatile (sometimes too versatile), are outgoing and interact wonderfully with people. They are inventive and excellent problem-solvers. Somebody else will have to do the labor because the Gemini person does the mental work rapidly and easily and then moves on to something else. The Gemini person is usually warm, impulsive and quite fickle in love affairs. They tire quickly of people, places and things. They're always looking for something new and exciting. Wonderful companions but indifferent spouses.

PHYSICAL ASPECTS

There is a tendency towards overexhaustion, and to problems connected with the shoulders, arms, lungs and nervous systems. The Gemini person should not be so careless about health, should observe moderation and try to control energy instead of scattering it. Gemini persons should work at stimulating jobs for happiness.

CANCER

People born under the sign of Cancer can be strongly influenced by their early home life. On one hand they can be powerful and extremely influential because with their strong will and tenacity they can literally move mountains. On the other hand they can also be extremely lazy and self-indulgent without an ambition in the world. Both types are extremely intelligent and highly original in their thinking. Both types can be warm, loving and excellent marriage material. However, there is a tendency to be extremely sensitive to real or imagined slights and hurts. Cancer persons can very easily use alcohol to drown hurts, fears and worries, or take to overeating.

PHYSICAL ASPECTS

There is a tendency to weakness in the stomach, breasts and elbow joints. Moderation in eating and an avoidance of alcohol is advised. Self-confidence and emotional stability can be achieved through the satisfaction of creative invention.

LEO

This is a magnificent sign. Persons born under this sign are truly regal. They are proud but magnanimous. They are honest and honorable in everything they do or say. Because they are this way they find it difficult to believe that everyone isn't. While they are swift to anger if hurt or misused, they are quick to forgive and forget. Leo people cannot function in menial positions, they are superb in executive positions and are quite wonderful with responsibility because they will truly and faithfully discharge each responsibility they are given.

PHYSICAL ASPECTS

There is a tendency to weakness in the Gall Bladder, Heart and Back but Leo's have tremendous recuperative powers. Moderation in all things is a must for Leo's. They also need to cultivate tact instead of blunt honesty with people.

VIRGO

Here is the true intellectual of the zodiac. Unlike the Gemini who is also intellectual but somewhat facile, the Virgo person really absorbs knowledge like a sponge, remembers and uses everything and makes major contributions. Virgos really know what it's all about and sometimes tend to criticize without rancor or pride but just because right is right. Virgos are usually quite reserved and unassuming and generally are not really and fully appreciated for the depth of knowledge that they possess. Virgos make marvelous mathematicians and can work alone (they prefer it) without need for supervision. They can be extremely tactful but really have little sympathy for others, are cool in love or marriage and cannot be possesed.

PHYSICAL ASPECTS

The tendency to weakness in the Abdomen and small intestines can lead to Digestive Disorders, Diarrhea, Constipation, Colitis, Hernia and Appendicitis. However, since most Virgos have a sense of balance in diet and tend to take care of their health, there is little to fear in these areas.

LIBRA

Here are the naturally well-bred people. Good taste and good manners are inherent to the Libra person. Although they are extremely fastidious (can't stand mess or dirt in people or in things), they are affectionate, sympathetic and kind. They need love and affection and are usually married or, if not married, have a steady companion. Libra people make superb art and music critics because their sense of proportion and balance is excellent. They also make excellent lawyers and judges because of a keen sense of justice. They will go to the ends of the earth to right a wrong or an injustice. Incidentally they are magnificent in sex which they raise to a fine art. They have trouble sometimes in arriving at a decision because they tend to see both sides equally and try to be completely fair to both sides.

PHYSICAL ASPECTS

There is a tendency to weakness in the lower back and the kidneys. Skin eruptions and headaches are also trouble areas. However, Libra people have excellent constitutions and recuperate quickly from illness and disease.

SCORPIO

This is the oddest sign on the zodiac. The Scorpio person is a true paradox in that the highest and lowest characteristics can be combined in one person. Regardless of looks, the Scorpio is sex appeal personified. Personal magnetism is always present and can be literally overpowering. You can be certain that Scorpio people get their way—always. They make magnificent friends and lovers but terrible enemies. When you wrong or wound a Scorpio—look out—retaliation is on its way, inexorably. When the higher type of Scorpio is present, the world benefits immeasurably in science, medicine and criminal detection. Scorpios are dedicated workers with boundless energy. When the lower type is present you have the master criminal—the arch-fiend and the master spy. As a lover Scorpio has no match for sheer passion but beware of jealousy—once aroused it can be devastating. Scorpios are extremely possessive.

PHYSICAL ASPECTS

Thre is a tendency to weakness in the pelvic area which includes the intestines, urinary and genitals. Scorpio people generally have marvelous recuperative powers however.

SAGITTARIUS

Here is the true aristocratic type. High spirited, impetuous and extremely refined. The true story book character—bold, proud and brave. Your general disposition is bright and cheerful. Oddly enough, although you will resent coarseness in other people, you are not a snob, but rather are truly democratic. You are friends with all people to whom you grant unlimited freedom—but you also insist upon full freedom for yourself. Your strongest asset is your uncanny intuition—it's always right. If you follow it you succeed in all things. If you ignore it, you fail. Marriage isn't for you, you treasure freedom too much. Small details bore you but the big picture enthralls you. Outdoors is your playground.

PHYSICAL ASPECTS

There is a tendency to weakness in the thighs, hips and tendons. Carelessness in these regard (coupled with your impetuous nature) can produce laziness. Because you're high strung you should guard against a breakdown.

CAPRICORN

People born under this sign usually have towering ambition. You have, in addition, all of the attributes that can lead to success. Like your sign (The Goat) you have the ability to leap over obstacles (and competitors) in your climb to the top. You have a strong sense of duty and responsibility although when you assume responsibility, you will sometimes have a tendency to complain about the burden. You are a true conservative and stick to the tried-and-true. What was good for your father is good enough for you. Your worst fault is a tendency to be over-righteous and convinced that you are always right. You also tend to be domineering, especially with your children. Your best arsenal is your iron constitution, nerves of stainless steel and endurance beyond belief.

PHYSICAL ASPECTS

There is a tendency towards Rheumatism, Arthritis and Neuralgia. This is compounded by your habit of brooding. Cheer up, avoid hypochondria and live to be well past 100.

AQUARIUS

This is the sign of the great humanitarians. They are noble, moderate and sound. People with this sign have a deep knowledge of human nature and a tolerance for human weakness. There is a scientific bent and a love of invention and new discoveries. There is usually a remarkable power of observation coupled with a strong intuitive sense that amounts to genius. People with this sign usually are uncanny in their ability to predict the future. They have a strong belief in the brotherhood of man and believe in the eventual world order in which peace and harmony will reign throughout the world and all mankind will be brothers.

PHYSICAL ASPECT

The overall aspects are very good with only a slight tendency to weakness in the calves, ankles and the fluid carrying vessels of the body, particularly the lymph glands. But because people in this sign are moderate in their habits and don't abuse their bodies, there is all indications of good health and long long life.

PISCES

This is the true psychic sign. People born under this sign are considerate, sensitive and highly intuitive. There is also a tendency towards a vivid imagination and to be highly suggestible. Although people in this sign appear to be idealistic they are, in reality, quite down to earth in solving problems or earning money. This is also the sign of the mystic and the religious. The Piscean is devoted to loved ones, sometimes overconcerned, overprotective. While you do many things you rarely do them for praise—but ingratitude causes deep hurts.

PHYSICAL ASPECTS

There is a tendency to trouble with the feet and excretory fluids of the body. Generally the health of the Pisceans is excellent but there is little power to resist disease. Proper diet, rest and moderation are keynotes to good health and long life.

Astrology offers other information of a health/medical nature. Astrologer Ruth Schwarz states "Never schedule an operation when the moon is full, unless there is a real emergency. Humans seem to bleed more heavily and uncontrollably at this time."

Are we really so closely affected by the stars?

Perhaps the above theory is totally erroneous. And yet, other disciplines, other fields of science are nibbling around the edges of theories just such as this one, concerning timing, human rhythmnicity and health.

Consider, for example, the so-called *circadian* rhythmn (from the Latin circa (around) dies (a day)). This inherent cycle appears over approximately a 24 hour period.

Skin temperature shows evidence of major change during the circadian rhythm.

Blood pressure, respiration and amino acid levels all change within the circadian cycle.

Patients in hospitals feel more pain during certain time periods rather than others.

Perhaps the astrologers know something the rest of us have long forgotten?

Certain facts seem to be emerging.

The central nervous system would appear to be affected by the frequencies of the moon and other planets which alter the body's electromagnetic field.

Tokyo doctor/astrologers have tested human blood and found that the composition varies in reaction to solar eclipses.

The celestial panorama holds some sort of undercover role . . . some pull or influence on us . . . or so the bits and pieces of fact would seem to indicate.

Perhaps in our lifetimes, medical science and the ancient art of astrology will merge in new knowledge and procuedures available to improve the quality and length of our lives!

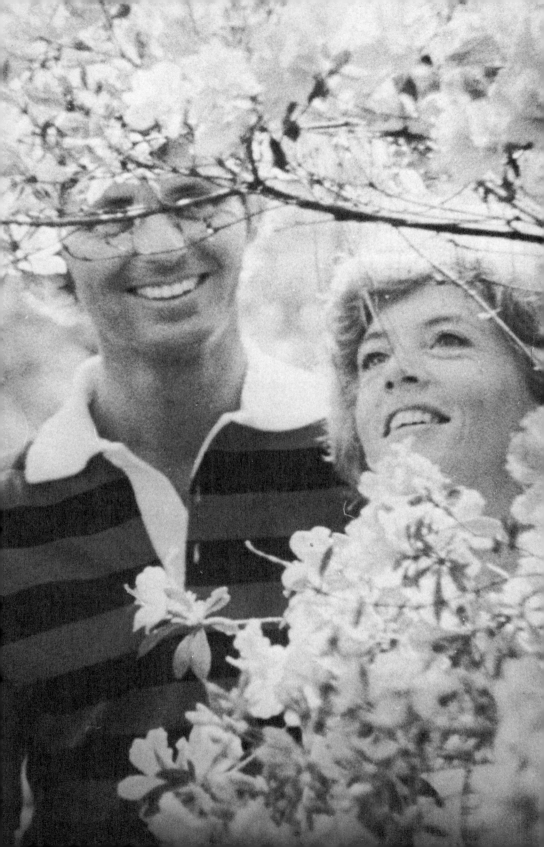

CHAPTER TEN

YOU CAN BE YOUNGER NOW

Sooner or later I'm going to die,
but I'm not going to retire.
　　　　　MARGARET MEAD
　　　　　(when she turned 75)

Margaret Mead is a remarkable woman. She is, at 75 as active and interested in life as she was at 30. Perhaps more so because she's so much more experienced. She is one of the world's most respected anthropologists, explorers and humanists. She has led a life of continuous action and change and, from the looks of it, will go on leading exactly that kind of life. It doesn't matter to Margaret Mead how long she lives. What matters is that she makes every day of her life count for something. She enjoys every day just as much, if not more so, than when she started out to become the leading anthropologist of our time.

There's a remarkable lesson in the example of healthy, interested, long life that she presents. It would be safe to say that every day is filled with challenges, experiences and new discoveries for her. *Just as it can be for you.* There is no reason why each and every day of your life can't be filled with excitement and discoveries. They'll be different than the ones that Margaret Mead discovers but that's because she's different from you. You are a unique person and therefore your excitement and your discoveries will be unique and different if you let them happen to you. If you do not retire from life but rather go out and embrace life with both hands.

Change is the key note to discovery. The slightest change in your daily routine can open new vistas, new avenues which may contain unique and wonderful surprises. Think about your daily routine. Is there some way you could change it? Even the very simple changes can make a big difference.
For example:

Do you drive to your shopping area? Take a bus for a change. Or call a taxi. Or, if it's close enough—walk.

Is there a museum or planetarium near you—one that you have never visited? Make a date with yourself to go. Spend an afternoon at either one—or both. Give yourself new insight.

Have you ever visited an art gallery? Make a date to visit one. Particularly if there's a 'one man show' going on.

How about making a date to take yourself to a concert? Or a musical? Perhaps a legitimate play?

Do you notice that I'm advising you to make a date with yourself—rather than with someone? That's because these should be your experiences—not yours and someone else's. Just yours. Because we're concerned with changes for *you*. There's no need to share every experience with someone. You don't read a book with someone. You read it by yourself.

Learn to do other things by yourself. Take a piece of paper and a pencil or pen and write down a list of things that you would enjoy doing by yourself. Try to make the list as uninhibited as possible. I mean, by that, don't allow considerations like money and time interfere with your desires. Just write down whatever you would like to do. Let's suppose 'travel' is on your mind. List everyone of the countries you would like to visit. It doesn't matter that you haven't got the money or the time to travel the way you would like to.

Now let's do something dramatic. Take that list of countries you want to visit to your local travel agent. Ask him what it would cost you to travel to those countries. Tell him you'd like some travel brochures about those countries. Take your brochures and your cost of travel information home with you. Study the brochures. Now think about this. If you have a steady job, a bank will (if you have no bad credit marks) lend you the money to travel. When is your vacation due? You could start saving money for additional expenses—then, when you're ready, you'll have travel and expense money. It would be a good idea to apply for your passport now because it can take up to six weeks to get one.

Is the prospect beginning to excite you? Of course it is. It should excite you because it's an exciting idea of a healthy change for you. A chance to do something that you've always wanted to do but never thought you'd have the time or money.

You can generate excitement with change—either actual or contemplated. That excitement can make you young again because that's part of being young—to be capable of excitement and expectation. So start thinking about changes you can make. Give yourself short and long-range goals.

Write some more changes you'd like to make on that list. How about your hairstyle? Why not change it? What about your clothes? Are you game for a new look—a new you?

Did you ever keep a TIME and MOTION INVENTORY? This is probably one of the most eyeopening adventures you can take. You only have to do it for one day in order to gain surprising insight into your life and the way you conduct it.

Just take a sheet of paper and, in bold letters print:

TIME AND MOTION

Date: _____

TIME	ACTIVITY
7:00 AM	_____
7:15	_____
7:30	_____
7:45	_____
8:00	_____

The idea is to make out the sheet the night before the day you will take inventory. Start the time with the time you generally wake up. Then set up the sheet for 15 minute periods from that time until the time you go to bed. Write down everything you do in each 15 minute period. If you do a lot—give yourself more space between time periods. Just remember, you must stop at each 15 minute period and write down exactly what you did. Don't scribble—try to be legible because you'll want to read it all later on. Take another piece of paper and cover what you write when you finish it—and don't peek the next time you start to write down your next 15 minutes. That way you'll have some surprises when you finish.

Incidentally—don't forget to record exactly what you eat during the day—whether it's at a mealtime or in between. That's part of your inventory too.

If you leave your house or apartment for something, then be sure to write down exactly what you did and how long it took you (how many 15 minute periods).

You can take this same kind of a list to work with you and do exactly the same thing and discover exactly how much actual work you do during the day and how much goofing off you do.

The idea of all this is to give you a realistic grip on your life and a definite way to change it for the better. When you have these inventories complete and ready to study you'll have actual knowledge of the patterns in your life—whether they're work, play or eating. You can change each of these areas.

Make certain of one thing—*whatever changes you make, there must be a commensurate reward that goes with it*. The reward can be tangible or intangible. For example, if you give up certain foods—like potato chips or candy—you can reward yourself with either an intangible (like the reminder of the weight you will lose and the nice new figure you'll have) or, if you can afford it, you can buy yourself a present—it can be a small one like a book—or gloves—maybe new shoes—but something that will provide you with a reward factor. Without reward of some kind you will tend to lose enthusiasm and fall back into your old bad habits and it will be worse because you'll suffer from loss of self esteem for your failure.

There's no joy in suffering the humiliation of a defeat by a cigarette, candy bar or a glass of beer or liquor. So learn to reward yourself for your efforts. Develop a sense of real appreciation of yourself, especially for any small changes you are able to make in your habits. *The idea is to reward yourself for what you have accomplished rather than to punish yourself for what you didn't manage to accomplish.* In addition to being a more pleasant way to behave, it's also more effective in helping yourself to achieve changes.

Remember that it's best to affect small successful changes rather than to attempt (and fail) to achieve big changes. Do your changes one step at a time and remember to take small steps because they're easier.

The major enemy of change is inertia—the tendency to let things remain as they are. One of the laws of the universe states: "The hardest part is to get started."

If you decide to give up smoking (which is a major change and loaded with stress) then get a jar or a can and put sixty or seventy cents in the pot for each pack of cigarettes you did not smoke. Do this at the end of the day. Watching that money amount up day after day will be one of the best rewards you can give yourself. It's the most noticeable. The next most noticeable thing is the fact that your cough will disappear. When the money reaches a certain point—buy yourself something with that money.

This type of reward pattern creates positive reinforcement of your original intention and desire. There is another type of good strong reinforcement which consists of a listing of all of the benefits that will result from the particular habit change that you have made in your lifestyle. Make the list as long as possible and then put it up in the kitchen or the bathroom.

Here's an example of a list made by a determined dieter. *Please note that the benefits listed are entirely realistic.*

YOUR MOTIVATION LIST

Here is an idea of the kind of list you should write:
1. I will look slimmer and younger.
2. My complexion will improve.
3. My clothes will fit better.
4. I'll be able to exercise easily.
5. People will compliment me for my appearance.
6. I'll feel more confidence in myself.

Your list could include these items or others you might think of. The main objective is to make a list of items that will give you incentive to continue towards your goals. Each item must be important to you. The more successful you are in finding items that motivate you, the better your list.

You should, as you go along, make a list of interim goals that you have reached and are aware of.

INTERIM GOALS—ACHIEVED

1. My waist is growing smaller.
2. I lost_____ pounds.
3. My clothes are fitting better.
4. I received 2 compliments today (date).

Remember, visible progress means self encouragement and reinforcement of your determination to continue.

ACCOMPLISHMENTS

1. I have eliminated desserts.
2. I am eating smaller portions of food.
3. I eat a soundly balanced, nutritious breakfast.
4. I am now chewing my food thoroughly.

This kind of a list is extremely valuable in providing the reward for achievement and further reinforcement of your desire to continue your program. It also provides visible evidence of your success in establishing positive patterns.

Another technique you can use to help reinforce your desire to continue is called 'chaining' which simply means chaining an undesirable action to your undesirable habit. It makes it more difficult to engage in your bad habit (such as smoking). For example, you might place your cigarettes in your car and lock the car door. Then place the keys to the car in an envelope. Next, take all the matches and cigarette lighters and put them in the cellar. Then, whenever you have the desire to smoke you must go to so much trouble that you may decide not to, at that time. The longer you go without smoking each time you have the urge, the sooner you will arrive at your major objective of giving them up altogether.

You can also try the reward/punishment idea. That is, whenever you want to smoke, make yourself do a disagreeable task that you can then link to the undesirable habit.

On the other hand you can link a pleasurable or agreeable action (watching a favorite TV show, for example) as a reward for not smoking during the program.

If you put your mind to it, you can eventually condition yourself to associate smoking with all undesirable and disagreeable things. You merely have to examine your regular habits, your likes and dislikes as well as your particular needs. If you set up a firm 'pairing' program and stick to it, you'll be amazed at how swiftly your basic conditioning relative to smoking will change.

Please remember the axiom: *All change produces stress.* That means you will need all the assistance you can get from your Alpha relaxation technique. Use it often. If you should suddenly feel tired, stop and rest. Fatigue is dangerous to the success of your self-improvement program.

You will find that your most vulnerable time comes when you are tired because that's when you are most likely to give in to an urge to nibble some candy, take a short drink or smoke that extra cigarette. Just remember that fatigue can cause you to fall back on old habits. It can also lead to some self-pity and dangerous thoughts like *"I've been so good, just one won't hurt me,"* or *"What would it hurt if I took one little piece of candy?"* or *"I'll smoke this one cigarette and then I won't smoke another one for three hours."*

Don't do it. You mustn't compromise or plea-bargain because as soon as you do, you're going to go right back into your bad, old habits again and there goes the program down the drain and it will be twice as hard to start it up again.

So stick to your guns, keep working at that program and remind yourself, at every step, that backsliding can mean a total disaster for the entire program, not just one part of it. Once you give in to a momentary weakness your entire morale starts falling apart and you begin to feel guilty and discouraged. This leads to further relaxation of your care and watchfulness. You then have strong doubts that you will succeed and as this conviction grows you begin to indulge yourself more and more.

Stay on the positive side. Keep reminding yourself of the rewards that your program will give you. Go over your list of interim achievements, then check out your progress to date. Dwell on the success of each item. Reinforce your desire to succeed with the program and, eventually, you will succeed in achieving everything you set out to do.

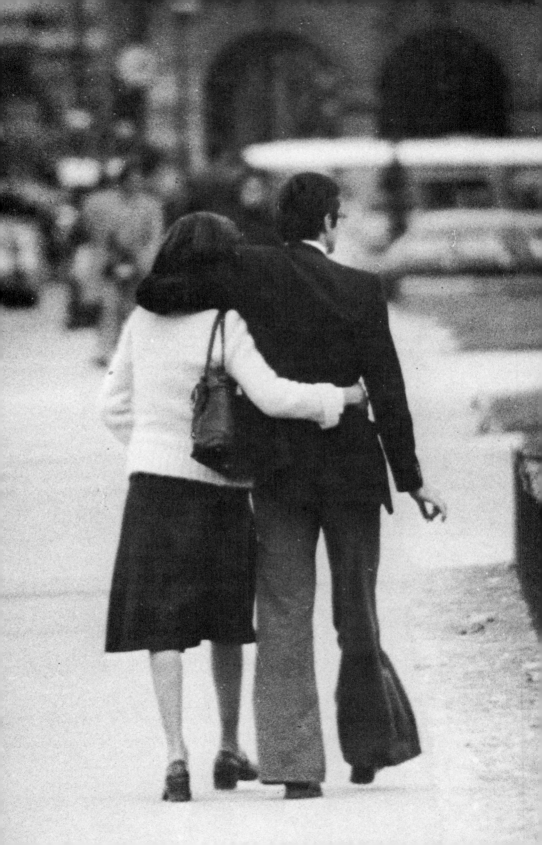

CONCLUSION

Life and living are each, in their own way, comparable to the production of a clear, pure note "A" by a major symphonic orchestra. That particular note, throughout the musical world, is always exactly 440 cycles per second, or—to put it in musical terms, "A" is the sixth tone in the scale of C major or the first tone in the scale of A minor.

All of the hundred odd musical instruments in the large orchestra are producing this single note, yet none of them will sound exactly alike because each instrument has uniquely different overtones. *No two instruments are exactly alike.*

Life, on this planet Earth is like that pure note "A"—it flows through every living thing and is the fixed harmonic note that we all vibrate to. Yet, every living thing on this planet Earth is uniquely different. The billions of people on this Earth produce individual overtones as they resonate to that living harmonic.

That particular 'resonating' is what we call 'living a life' and just as each musician's task is to resonate harmonically in accordance with the laws of harmonics; just so do we humans have to resonate in harmony with the life force that courses through our bodies.

When our bodies are 'in tune' with our life force harmonic we are healthy and filled with the joy of living and being. When we are not in tune, there is discord and disease and a joyless juiceless existence which we seek to end. We can seek that end abruptly or stretch it out over a decade or more of misery.

YOU CHOOSE

The choice is always ours—at any point in our life we may choose harmony or discord. No one forces the choice upon us. No one forces you to be an up-tight, compulsive 'work-a-holic' rushing through each working day at breakneck speed; then lying awake half the night worrying about tomorrow's problems. No one forces you to abuse your body with cigarettes, liquor, excessive amounts of coffee and junk food.

No one can really force you to do anything you do not want to do. Only you. You are in complete charge of yourself. You and you alone are responsible for your life.

Now that you've read this book you no longer can plead ignorance because you know the facts of life as they exist. You know that it is physically possible to live to 100 and beyond. The people of Transcaucasia, of Hunza, of Vilcambama, Ecuador are doing it right now. They're living and enjoying life well past 125 years of age. You can, too.

All of the basic knowledge you need to begin living a healthy and happier life has been presented to you in this book. You can change, if you want to. You *must* change if you want to extend your life in addition to making it a happier one.

Some change is inevitable.

You are a changed person right now. In addition to the many continuous changes that have taken place in your body since you first began to read this book, there is another, more subtle change that has taken place within you.

You are more familiar now with the working of your body and, even more importantly, the *needs* of your body. You are aware of the substances you must obtain to satisfy your body's daily needs; as well as the substances that you must avoid if your body is to become well and healthy again.

Remember this: regardless of your age, regardless of the current physical condition of your body, it can be restored to glowing health *if you really want it to be restored.*

The prime requirement is your attitude.

You must become determined to take command of yourself in a positive instead of a negative way. Re-evaluate yourself. Think positively about yourself; about your skills, your talents, your essential being. Learn to love, admire and respect yourself and then you will be capable of loving, admiring and respecting other people and they, in turn, will react the same way to you.

Treat your body with the same respect and consideration you give to your car. You wouldn't dream of dumping sand or other abrasives into your crankcase, along with the motor oil. When you hear strange noises under the hood you take your car to a garage for a checkup. You see that it has a 'tune-up' at regular intervals. You check the tires to see that they're properly inflated. In essence, you treat your car with intelligent care and consideration *because you want it to last.*

If you give your body the same care and consideration it will also last—much longer than any car will. A healthy, well-tuned body will also give you a great deal more pleasure and deep happiness. And the odd part about it, the cost of the upkeep of a well-tuned body is nominal. In fact, you can actually save money while you're doing it. Just by eliminating liquor and cigarettes you can give yourself a boost in take-home pay.

The Alpha state, which you now know how to accomplish, costs you absolutely nothing, and yet it can do more to restore your body and mind than all the drugs and therapy in the world. Once you learn how to create the Alpha state, at will, nothing that happens in the world can invade your calm. You will have become invulnerable to the stress and frustration induced by hectic pace of modern business. Even more importantly, you will have a calming effect on those about you, whether it's at home or at work. You will become the center of calm, the focal point of logic and reason in any crisis.

Now, at this point, I would suggest that you make a definite decision with regard to the rest of your life. Make a decision to begin to live as you were meant to live. Make a decision to begin immediately to restore your body and mind to complete health through a series of easily obtainable objectives.

Take a piece of paper and write in large capital letters;

I AM GOING TO BEGIN TO CHANGE MY LIFE NOW!

Then say it aloud. Get up from your chair and begin to walk up and down and say it aloud with determination and belief.

Keep saying it, keep walking back and forth and as you do, an astonishing thing will begin to happen. You will find yourself growing taller as your head comes up and your posture improves.

Now, even more amazing, is the change you will begin to perceive in your inner being. There will be a stirring and a tingling at the back of your neck. You will feel a surge of power sweeping through you from the top of your head to the tips of your toes.

Each time you repeat that determination it will become much stronger and you will notice a change in your voice as the belief and strength grows inside you. A dynamic change is taking place inside you. A change that will grow and continue to grow with each passing day. Now, while this change is taking place, sit down and write this note to yourself:

HERE ARE THE CHAPTERS
I MUST REVIEW:

1. **Chapter Two: The Enemies of Long Life**
You must be fully aware of these enemies if you are going to overcome them. Study this chapter—take notes.

2. **Chapter Three: Learning About Your Body**
Become thoroughly familiar with the key features of your body; become conscious of the needs of your heart, your lungs, your liver and your kidneys. Pay attention to your bowel movements—learn to give yourself that vitally important enema.

3. **Chapter Four: Lifestyle and Life Expectancy**
This is a critically important chapter because it represents an area of your life that you can do something about immediately. You *must* do something about your lifestyle as quickly as possible.

4. **Chapter Five: What You Eat is How You Age**
If you read no other chapter in this book but this one, you will lose a great deal, but you would still benefit immensely from the vital material in this chapter.

5. **Chapter Six: How To Live Longer, Look Younger**
Here, in essence, is what you really want to do. Read exactly how to do it simply, easily and without spending a penny on equipment or lessons.

6. **Chapter Seven: Sexual Activity and Long Life**
   This not only tells you that it's possible to have both long life and a continuous sex life—it also tells how to do it.

7. **Chapter Eight: Choice of Stress or Serenity**
   This is the chapter that can, almost from the moment you put the instructions to work, will change your life for the better and keep on changing it each day of your life.

8. **Chapter Nine: Using Astrology to Stay Young**
   Here, in this chapter, in simple terms, are basic facts about yourself that you can use to your advantage. You don't have to believe in astrology. Just read about yourself and decide whether or not it makes sense.

9. **Chapter Ten: You Can Be Younger Right Now**
   If you actually walked around making your new decision aloud—you should already feel younger. Read this chapter again (plus this Conclusion) and see if you don't feel younger and healthier right now. It really works!

Please remember that all change causes stress. Even the decision to make a change will cause a certain amount of stress. This is not always a bad thing as long as you use up the products of stress. That's why I asked you to walk up and down while making your decision a verbal message. That way, you used up the materials your body produces as soon as any stress condition arises.

Always keep that in mind. Change causes stress—stress produces a package of energy that must be consumed. If you are shocked or suddenly angered—remember the package of energy and use it. Just stiffen your arms or legs or flex your hands rapidly and the products of stress will flow to those muscles and be used to good effect.

Develop the power of the Alpha state as quickly as possible. Practice placing yourself in an Alpha state at every opportunity. It should become almost a conditioned reflex and you will find that you are armored against the stupidity and injustice of this world and can approach any crisis with a clear and objective mind. You will also be a calming influence in crisis.

Finally you should think of the changes that you are going to make in your life as deposits in a bank account of life. If you make deposits regularly each day, regardless of the size of the deposit, your account will grow and flourish.

Give yourself short term, easily obtainable goals and your achievements will encourage you to greater effort. Start out slowly and gradually step up the pace and remember— moderation is the keynote to whatever you do, whether it's eating, exercising or making changes.

If you should encounter any problems that you think I might be able to help you with, please write to me care of the publisher. I promise you a quick response.

Good luck and much joy in your new life.

WEIGHT

CONTROL

SUPPLEMENT

3000 Different foods evaluated

TABLE OF CONTENTS

BETTER NUTRITION AND DIET

The principle of better nutrition and diet is quite simple. We have divided food into three basic categories. In the first category, you can have all you want. This is the "green or go category." Your body will tell you when you've had enough carrots, for instant. However, tomatoes have more calories and although they are nutritious and healthful, you must learn to limit and balance them in your diet.

Tomatoes are therefore, part of the second category—the yellow or "caution" category. This is the classification you must watch carefully. Count up the points as you're planning a meal, keep the calorie count under 1000.

The third category is red or "stop." Quite simply, food in this category should never be eaten. They provide you with far too little nutrition for their high caloric content.

So start putting this booklet to good use today. You can have anything you like in green—don't even bother counting. But when you get that craving for something, and it's in the red, swap it for something as satisfying in the yellow. But watch out! Don't go over a hundred!

After you have reached your desired body weight, you may increase your caloric intake until you find the number of calories it takes to maintain your desired weight.

HINTS ON NUTRITION AND HEALTH

1. In addition to watching your calories, you should also watch the protein content of your food. Every human being needs protein every single day to be truly healthful. Protein is the basic building block for cell growth and renewal. Try to eat as much protein as possible within your calorie limitation each day. Chicken and fish are excellent sources of protein.

2. Take a high potency vitamin-mineral pill at least once a day and if your doctor thinks it is satisfactory, with

each meal. Be sure you select a vitamin-mineral which has all the basic nutrition requirements which have been proven to be needed by man.

3. Be sure to eat a good breakfast. Many people fall into the trap of not eating a good breakfast and fooling themselves by saying. "Well, I am going to save a bunch of calories." You need to wake up your system and to break your fast. This is the meaning of the word breakfast. Breakfast is probably the most important meal of the day.

4. Chew your food slowly and completely. Don't wolf your food down. Allow yourself to experience the complete food sensation.

5. Try small portions. For those of us who travel on airlines, we have experienced that small portions are really quite satisfactory. Even if they may not be the most tasteful food, they are satisfactory. Try to use smaller plates and utensils. We can in essence trick the subconscious mind into satisfaction by cleaning our plate, but by cleaning a smaller plate.

Remember, as we said before, the subconscious mind deals in generalities and it, therefore, will not be able to distinguish between an 8 inch plate and a 6½ inch plate.

6. Try to spend at least 10 minutes doing some physical exercises like calisthenics or swimming every

day. Try to use your body regularly, whenever possible. Walk instead of ride, take the stairs instead of the elevator.

7. Don't eat at night for a period of three hours before going to sleep. These calories are likely to be deposited in your rump and tummy.

8. Try each day to have some foods from the vegetable category, the fruit category and the milk and cheese category, as well as the meat and fish category and the green category. This is what is meant by a balanced nutrition. Do not take all your calories in the form of steak or in the form of dairy products but vary your caloric intake.

9. Know what food you are addicted to. Try to determine what stimuli, visual, auditory or smells stimulate your desire to eat.

10. Above all, be aware of eating. Wake up. Don't eat unconsciously, but consciously plan your eating so as to live a healthy and more slimming life.

11. Eat carefully when you eat out at a restaurant. Study the menu and count the calories just as cautiously as you would at home.

12. Once you've reached your desired weight, you can increase your calorie content, but remember, thin is in.

	unit	calories
Pouilly Fuisse (B&G, import)	2 oz	40
Red Burgundy (Italian Swiss, dom.)	2 oz	43
Chianti (Italian Swiss, dom.)	2 oz	43
Rhine (Italian Swiss, dom.)	2 oz	43
Chablis (Cruse & Fils Freres, import)	2 oz	43
Champagne (Mumm's, import)	2 oz	44
Chianti (Gancia, import)	2 oz	44
Red Burgundy (B & G, import)	2 oz	46
Y Rose (Taylor, dom.)	2 oz.	46
Claret (Taylor, dom.)	2 oz	46
Liebfraumilch (Dienard, import)	2 oz	46
Sparkling Burgundy (Taylor, dom.)	2 oz	52
Champagne (Korbel, dom.)	2 oz	52
Red Bordeaux (Chanson Pere & Fils)	2 oz	54
White Bordeaux (Chateau Olivier, import)	2 oz	54
Sauterne (Gold Seal, dom.)	2 oz	54
Beer (Gablinger)	8 oz	64
All distilled spirits with 80 proof	1 oz	67
Vermouth (Lejon, dry, dom.)	2 oz	68
All distilled spirits with 86 proof	1 oz	72
Vermouth (C&P, dry, import)	2 oz	74
All distilled spirits with 90 proof	1 oz	75
Brandy (ginger, 70 proof)	1 oz	75
Creme de cassis (35 proof)	2 oz	79
Sherry (Dry Sack, import)	2 oz	80
Apricot Brandy (71 proof)	1 oz	81
All distilled spirits with 100 proof	1 oz	83
Sloe gin (66 proof)	1 oz	85
Vermouth (Noilly Prat, sweet, import)	2 oz	88
R Vermouth (Taylor, dom.)	2 oz	88
Blackberry brandy (70 proof)	1 oz	100
Cherry brandy (70 proof)	1 oz	100
Creme de cacao (54 proof)	1 oz	101
Beer (Pabst Blue Ribbon)	8 oz	102
Beer (Shlitz)	8 oz	103
Beer (Budweiser)	8 oz	105
Ale	8 oz	106
Beer (Schaefer)	8 oz	106
Beer (Michelob)	8 oz	107
Beer (Carling's)	8 oz	108
Beer (Rheingold)	8 oz	110
Anisette (56 proof)	1 oz	111
Benedictine (86 proof)	1 oz	112
Creme de menthe (60 proof)	1 oz	112
Malt liquor (Country Club)	1 oz	115

BISCUITS

		calories
Buttermilk (Pillsbury Extra lights	1	55
Ballard Oven Ready	1	60
Pillsbury Buttermelts	1	60
Pillsbury Country Style	1	60
Y Baking Powder (Pillsbury Tenderflake)	1	60
Buttermilk (Ballard)	1	60
Buttermilk (Hungry Jack Extra Rich)	1	60
Hungry Jack Flaky	1	80
Baking Powder (1869) Brand)	1	80
R Buttermilk (1869 Brand)	1	80
Buttermilk (Hungry Jack Flaky)	1	85
Hungry Jack Butter Tastin	1	90
Hungry Jack Fluffy	1	90

		calories
Buttermilk (1869 Brank Heat n' Serve)	1	95
R Baking Powder (1869 Brand Heat n' Serve)	1	100
1869 Brand Butter Tastin	1	115

BREAD

		calories
Rye (Pepp. Farm Party)	1 slice	15
Pumpernickel (Pepp. Farm Party)	1 slice	20
Gluten (Thomas Glutogen)	1 slice	30
White (Arnold's Melba)	1 slice	40
Rye (Arnold's Diet Slice)	1 slice	45
Wheat, Whole (Arnold's Melba)	1 slice	45
Protein (Thomas' Protogen)	1 slice	45
White (Pepp. Farm Very Thin Sliced)	1 slice	45
White (Thomas' Rite-Diet)	1 slice	50
Profile Dark	1 slice	55
Rye (Wonder	1 slice	55
Wheat, Whole, 100% (Thomas) 16 oz. loaf	1 slice	55
Profile Light	1 slice	60
Rye, Beefsteak (Wonder Family)	1 slice	60
Y Wheat, Whole 100% (Wonder)	1 slice	60
Cinnamon-Raisin (Thomas)	1 slice	60
Cinnamon-Raisin (Wonder)	1 slice	60
White (Thomas 16 oz loaf)	1 slice	60
White (Wonder Daffodil)	1 slice	60
Rye, Sprouted (Pepp. Farm)	1 slice	65
Wheat (Buttertop Home Pride)	1 slice	65
Wheat (Wonder)	1 slice	65
Wheat, Cracked (Wonder)	1 slice	65
Wheat, Sprouted (Pepp. Farm)	1 slice	65
Wheat, Whole (Arnold's Brick Oven)	1 slice	65
Wheat, Whole (Arnold's Brick Oven-Sm Family)	1 slice	65
Wheat. Whole (Pepp. Farm)	1 slice	65
Wheat, Whole, 100% (Thomas) 29 oz loaf	1 slice	65
Wheat, Germ (Pepp. Farm)	1 slice	65
White (Arnold's Brick Oven Sm. Family)	1 slice	65
Corn & Mollasses, (Pepp. Farm)	1 slice	70
Oatmeal (Pepp. Farm)	1 slice	70
Wheat, Craked (Pepp. Farm)	1 slice	70
White (Arnold's Soft Sandwich)	1 slice	70
White (Buttertop Home Pride)	1 slice	70
White (Pep. Farm Sandwich)	1 slice	70
White (Thomas) 29 oz loaf	1 slice	70
White (Wonder)	1 slice	70
Nat Health (Arnold)	1 slice	75
Seven Grain (Arnold)	1 slice	75
White, (Pepp. Farm Eng. Tea Loaf)	1 slice	75
R Brown, Canned (B&M)	½ slice	80
Brown, with Raisins	½ slice	80
Honey (Pepp. Farm Family)	1 slice	80
Pumpernickel (Pepp. Fram Family)	1 slice	80
Rye, Beefsteak (Wonder)	1 slice	80
White (Pepp. Farm Large)	1 slice	80
Rye (Pepp. Farm Family)	1 slice	85
Rye, Jewish (Arnold)	1 slice	85
Rye, Seedless (Pepp. Farm)	1 slice	85
White (Pepp. Farm Toasting White)	1 slice	85
French (Pepp. Farm)	1 1" slice	90
Italian (Pepp. Farm)	1 1" slice	90

BUTTER AND OILS

Y	Margarine, Imitation (Diet Mazola)	1 tbsp	50
	Butter, Whipped	1 tbsp	70
	Margarine, Soft (Nucoa)	1 tbsp	90
	Butter	1 tbsp	100
	Margarine (Mazola)	1 tbsp	100
	Margarine (Nucoa)	1 tbsp	100
	Margarine, Unsalted (Mazola)	1 tbsp	100
R	Oil, Safflower (Kraft)	1 tbsp	120
	Oil, Vegetable (Kraft)	1 tbsp	120
	Oil, Corn (Mazola)	1 tbsp	125
	Butter, Whipped	¼ cup	270
	Butter	¼ cup	405
	Lard	¼ cup	465
	Oil, Salad	¼ cup	485

CAKES

Date Nut Cake (Thomas')	1 sixth	90
Coffee Cake, Cinnamon (Pillsbury Country)	12"x4" pc	105
Coffee Cake, Cinnamon (Pepperidge Farm Twist)	one sixth	175
Coffee Cake, Apple (Morton)	one sixth	195
Pound Cake (Morton)	one sixth	205
R — Chocolate, German (Morton)	one sixth	21)
Coffee Cake, Pecan (Morton Danish Twist)	one sixth	230
Coffe Cake, Cinnamon (Morton Meltaway)	one sixth	250
Chocolate Fudge (Pepperidge Farm)	one sixth	320
Yellow (Pepperidge Farm)	one sixth	320
Coconut (Pepperidge Farm)	one sixth	330
Devils Food (Pepperidge Farm)	one sixth	330
Vanilla (Pepperidge Farm)	one sixth	330

CAKES, SNACK

Brownies, (Hostess), 2 pkg	1	100
HoHo, 2/pks.	1	105
HoHo, Family Carton	1	105
Cupcakes, Devils Food (Hostess), Family Carton	1	125
Twinkies, Family Carton	1	130
Cupcakes, Orange (Hostell), Family Carton	1	135
Snoballs	1	135
Twinkies, 2/pkg		
R — Cupcakes, Orange (Hostess), 2/pkg	1	150
Cupcakes, Devils Food (Hostess), 2/pkg	1	160
Ding Dong, Dark Chocolate, Family Carton	1	165
Ding Dong, Milk Chocolate Family Carton	1	165
Big Wheels, 2/pkg	1	170
Ding Dong, Dark Chocolate 2/pkg	1	170
Ding Dong, Milk Chocolate, 2/pkg	1	170
Suzy Q	1	230

CANDIES

G	Sugarless Bubble Gum (Estee)	1 pkg	3½
Y	Assorted Gum Drops (Estee)	4 candies	12
R	Kisses (Hershey's)	1	25
	Estee-ets Plain	6 candies	40

	Peanut Butter Cups (Resse's)	1	135
	Hershey-ets	34 (1 oz)	140
	Chocolate with Almonds, Bar (Hershey's)	1.3 oz	200
R	Krackel, Bar	1.4 oz	210
	Chocolate, Bar (Hershey's)	1.4 oz	220
	Special Dark, Bar	1.4 oz	220
	Rally, Bar	1.8 oz	260
	Mr. Goodbar, Bar	1.8 oz	280

CEREAL—COLD & HOT

	Quaker Puffed Rice	1 cup	45
	Kellog's Special K	1 cup	70
	Kix	1 cup	75
Y	Corn Flakes (Kellogg's)	1 cup	85
	Honeycomb Sweet Crisp	1 cup	85
	Cheerios	1 cup	88
	Corn Flakes (General Mills)	1 cup	88
	Total	1 cup	88
	Bran Flakes, 40 (Kellogg's)	1 cup	95
	Puffed Rice (State Fair)	1 cup	100
	Puffed Rice (Sunland)	1 cup	100
	Puffed Rice (Whiffs)	1 cup	100
	Malt-O-Meal, Quick	1 cup	105
	Malt-O-Meal, Chocolate	1 cup	105
	Apple Jacks	1 cup	110
	Baron Von Redberry	1 cup	110
	Boo Berry	1 cup	110
	Buc Wheats	1 cup	110
	Cocoa Puffs	1 cup	110
	Corn Chex	1 cup	110
	Corn Flakes (Ralston	1 cup	110
	Count Chocula	1 cup	110
	Crisp Rice	1 cup	110
	Franken Berry	1 cup	110
	Frosty O's	1 cup	110
	Great Honey Crunches, rice	1 cup	110
	Great Honey Crunches, wheat	1 cup	110
	Kaboom	1 cup	110
	Lucky Charms	1 cup	110
	Oatmeal Instant (Quaker)	1 cup	110
	Post Toasties Corn Flakes	1 cup	110
	Product 19	1 cup	110
R	Alpha-Bits, sugar frosted	1 cup	113
	Crispy Critters	1 cup	115
	All Bran	1 cup	115
	Fruit Loops	1 cup	120
	Grits Instant (Quaker)	1 cup	120
	Oatmeal with apples & cinnamon (Quaker)	1 cup	120
	Puffa Puffa Rice	1 cup	120
	Farina with water & Salt (Pillsbury)	1 cup	130
	Granola, regular (Gen. Mills)	1 cup	130
	Granola, cinnamon (Gen. Mills)	1 cup	130
	Pebbles, Cocoa	1 cup	130
	Pebbles, fruity	1 cup	130
	Pep	1 cup	135
	100s Bran (Nabisco)	1 cup	140
	Cap'n Crunch	1 cup	145
	Cocoa Krispies	1 cup	145
	Sugar frosted corn flakes (Kellogg)	1 cup	145
	King Vitamin	1 cup	145
	40s Bran Flakes (Post)	1 cup	150
	Grape Nuts Flakes	1 cup	160
	Oatmeal with raisins & spice (Quaker)	1 pkt	160

(G)=Green (Y)=Yellow (R)=Red

	Life (Quaker)	1 cup	165
	Oat flakes, fortified (Post)	1 cup	165
	Pink Panther Flakes	1 cup	175
	Oatmeal with maple & brown sugar	1 cup	180
	Bran Buds	1 cup	210
	H-O Oats (instant, quick, old fashioned	1 cup dry	260
R	Whole Wheat (Pettyjohn)	1 cup uncooked	300
	Farina with milk & salt (Pillsbury)	1 cup	310
	Quaker Oats (quick & old fashioned)	1 cup uncooked	330
	Oats (Ralston-Purina)	1 cup	330
	Ralston (regular & instant)	1 cup	440
	Farina (Quaker	1 cup uncooked	600
	Farina (H-O)	1 cup uncooked	640

CHEESE

	Cottage (uncreamed)	1 oz	21
	Cottage (creamed)	1 oz	33
	Riccotta, moist (Borden)	1 oz	42
	Meunster (Gammolost diet)	1 oz	45
	Cheddar (skimmed milk)	1 oz	45
	Cream, imitation (Philadelphia)	1 oz	50
	Spread, Imitation (Kraft)	1 oz	50
	Neufchatel (Kraft calorie wise)	1 oz	70
	Mozzarella (Frigo	1 oz	79
Y	Spread (Velveeta)	1 oz	80
	Camember (dom)	1 oz	82
	Gouda (Borden	1 oz	86
	American (cheese food)	1 oz	90
	Kraft Super Blend (cheese food)	1 oz	92
	Hickory Smoke (Smokelle Cheese food)	1 oz	93
	Provolone (Borden)	1 oz	93
	Bonbel Brand (round)	1 oz	94
	Sharp (Kraft cheese food)	1 oz	97
	Cream (Philadelphia)	1 oz	100
	Limburger	10z	100
	Monterey Jack (Kraft natural	1 oz	100
	Swiss (natural)	1 oz	100
	Swiss (processed)	1 oz	100
	Brick (Kraft natural)	1 oz	104
	Edam (Kraft)	1 oz	105
R	Parmesan (Kraft	1 oz	107
	American (processed)	1 oz	110
	Blue	1 oz	110
	Cheddar (dom.)	1 oz	110
	Cheddar (natural)	1 oz	110
	Colby (natural	1 oz	110
	Gruyere (Kraft)	1 oz	110
	Roquefort	1 oz	110
	Swiss (dom.)	1 oz	110
	Parmesan (grated)	1 oz	130

COFFEE

G	Ground (Maxwell House)	6 fl oz	2
	Ground (Sanka)	6 fl oz	2
	Ground (Yuban)	6 fl oz	2
	Instant (Maxwell House)	6 fl oz	4
	Instant (Sanka)	6 fl oz	4
	Instant (Sanka)	6 fl oz	4
G	Instant (Yuban)	6 fl oz	4
	Freeze-dried (Maxim)	6 fl oz	4
	Freeze-dried (Sanka)	6 fl oz	4
Y	Postum (Cereal Beverage), Instant	1c	15

CONDIMENTS

	Sweet Magic	1 tsp.	0
	Sugar Twin	1 tsp.	1½
	Sweet 'n Low	1 pkt.	3
	Olives, Green, Medium	1	5
	Olives, Ripe	1 sm	6
		1 lg	9
G	Pickles, Dill	1(3¾"x¾")	8
	Tomato Catsup (Tillie Lewis Tasti Diet)	1 tbsp.	8
	Pickles, Dill, sliced	½ cup	9
	Mustard with Horseradish	1 tbsp.	10
	Pickle Relish, Sweet	1 tbsp.	12
	Soy Sauce	1 tbsp.	12
	Pickles, Sweet, Gherkin	1(2½"x¾")	22
Y	Pickles, Bread and Butter (Fanning's)	½ cup	60
	Tartar Sauce (Hellman's)	1 tbsp.	70

COOKIES

Y	Vanilla cookies (De Boles Dietetic)	1	13
	Arrowroot Biscuit (National)	1	20
	Biscos	1	20
	Cardiff (Pepperidge Farm)	1	20
	Nilla Wafers	1	20
	Social Tea Biscuit	1	20
	Ginger Snaps (Nabisco Old Fashion)	1	20
	Graham Crackers (Honey Maid)	1	30
	Graham Crackers (Nabisco)	1	30
	Lisbon (Pepperidge Farm)	1	30
	Molasses Crisp (Pepperidge Farm)	1	30
	Orleans (Pepperidge Farm)	1	30
	Bordeaux (Pepperidge Farm)	1	35
	Gingerman (Pepperidge Farm)	1	35
	Naples (Pepperidge Farm)	1	35
	Peanut Creme	1	35
	Pirouette, Lemon (Pepperidge Farm)	1	35
R	Piroutette, Original (Pepperidge Farm)	1	35
	Pirouette, Chocolate Laced (Pepperidge Farm)	1	40
	Shortbread (Lorna Doone)	1	40
	Brussels (Pepperidge Farm)	1	45
	Chewy Almond (Pillsbury	1	45
	Marquisette (Pepperidge Farm)	1	45
	Brown Sugar (Pepperidge Farm)	1	50
	Chocolate Chip (Pepperidge Farm)	1	50
	Cinnamon Sugar (Pepperidge Farm)	1	50
	Cinnamon Sugar (Pillsbury)	1	50
	Fudge Chip (Pepperidge Farm)	1	50
	Irish Oatmeal (Pepperidge Farm)	1	50
	Oreo	1	50
	Peanut Butter, Chocolate Chip (Pillsbury)	1	50
	Apple Cinnamon (Pillsbury)	1	55

Brownie, Chocolate Nut (Pepperidge Farm)	1	55
Butterscotch Nut (Pillsbury)	1	55
Chips Ahoy!	1	55
Chocolate Chip (Pillsbury)	1	55
Fig Newtons	1	55
Graham Crakers, Chocolate (Nabisco)	1	55
Mallomars	1	55
Oatmeal, Chocolate Chip (Pillsbury)	1	55
Oatmeal Raisin (Pepperidge Farm)	1	55
Peanut Butter (Pillsbury)	1	55
Sugar (Pepperidge Farm)	1	55
Sugar (Pillsbury)	1	55
Swiss Style Chocolate Chunk (Pillsbury)	1	55
Venice (Pepperidge Farm)	1	55
R Lemon Nut Crunch (Pepperidge Farm)	1	60
Oatmeal, Raisin (Pillsbury)	1	60
Milano (Pepperidge Farm)	1	65
Fudge Brownies (Pillsbury)	1 sq	70
Nutter Butter	1	70
Oatmeal (Nabisco)	1	75
Shortbread (Pepperidge Farm)	1	75
Dresden (Pepperidge Farm)	1	80
Mint Milan (Pepperidge Farm)	1	80
Capri (Pepperidge Farm)	1	85
Nassau (Pepperidge Farm)	1	85
Rochelle (Pepperidge Farm)	1	85
Rochelle (Pepperidge Farm)	1	85
Tahiti (Pepperidge Farm)	1	85
Lido (Pepperidge Farm)	1	95

CRACKERS

Goldfish Cheddar Cheese (Pepperidge Farm)	1	3
Goldfish Parmesan Cheese (Pepperidge Farm)	1	3
Goldfish Pizza (Pepperidge Farm)	1	3
Goldfish, Pretzel (Pepperidge Farm)	1	3
Goldfish, Sesame Garlic (Pepperidge Farm)	1	3
Soup and Oyster (Nabisco Dandy)	1	3
Cheese (Nabisco Nips)	1	5
Thins Wheat (Nabisco)	1	9
R Animal (Nabisco Barnum's)	1	10
Arti-Nugget STix	1	10
Sociables (Nabisco)	1	10
Thins, Bacon-Flavored (Nabisco)	1	10
Saltine (Nabisco Premium)	1	12
Ritz (Nabisco)	1	15
Thins, Cheese, Toasted (Pepperidge Farm)	1	15
Thins, Onion, Toasted (Pepperidge Farm)	1	15
Thins, Rye, Toasted Pepperidge Farm)	1	15
Thins, White, Toasted (Pepperidge Farm)	1	15
Escort (Nabisco)	1	20

Triscuit (Nabisco)	1	20
Ry Krisp	1	25
R Ry Krisp, Seasoned	1	30
Zwieback (Nabisco)	1	30
Ry Krisp, Family Size	¼ lg sq	45
Ry Krisp, Seasoned, Family Size	¼ lg sq	50

CREAM

Regular and Whipped	1 oz	110
Half and Half	1c	320
	1 tbsp	20
Sour Cream, Imitation	1c	440
	1 tbsp	20
R Sour Cream	1c	485
	1 tbsp	25
Light, Coffee or Table	1c	510
	1 tbsp	30
Whipping, Light	1c	720
	1 tbsp	45
Whipping, Heavy	1c	840
	1 tbsp	60

CREAMERS, NON DAIRY

Coffee-Mmate	1 tsp	11
Y Coffee-mate	1 pkt (3 grams)	17
Coffee-mate	1 fl oz	33

DRIED FRUIT

Apricots, Dried, Uncooked (Del Monte)	10 med halved	90
Prunes, Dried, Uncooked (Del Monte)	2 oz	120
Prunes, Moist-Pak with Pits (Del Monte)	2 oz	120
Apples, Evaporated, Uncooked (Del Monte)	2 oz	140
Apricots, Dried, Uncooked (Del Monte)	2 oz	140
Peaches, Dried, Uncooked (Del Monte)	2 oz	40
Prunes, Dried, Pitted (Del Monte)	2 oz	140
R Pears, Dried, Uncooked (Del Monte)	2 oz	150
Raisins, Muscat (Del Monte)	2 oz	165
Raisins, Golden Seedless (Del Monte)	2 oz	175
Raisins, Thompson Seedless (Del Monte)	2 oz	175
Apples, Dried, Cooked, Unsweetened	1c	200
Peaches, Dried, Cooked, Unsweetened	1c with liq	210
Pears, Dried, Cooked, Unsweetened	1c with liq	320
Currants (Del Monte)	1c	380
Peaches, Dried, Uncooked	1c	420
Pears, Dried, Uncooked	1c	480

EGGS

	Large, White Only	1	18
Y	Large, Yolk Only	1	60
	Large, Whole	1	80
	Egg Beaters	1	90
R	Large, Fried	1	100
	Large, Scrambled with Milk and Table Fat	1	110

ENTREES, CANNED, FROZEN

	Stew, chicken (B&M)	1 cup	130
	Turkey, Sliced in Gravy (Morton House)	1 can (4 1/6 oz)	140
	Beef, Patties and Burgundy Sauce (Morton House)	1 can	155
	Beef, Patties and Mexican Brand (Morton House)	1 can	155
	Salisbury Steak and Mushroom Gravey (Morton House)	1 can (4 1/6 oz)	160
	Patties and Italian Brand Sauce (Morton House)	1 can	170
	Meat Loaf in Gravy (Morton House)	1 can (4 1/6 oz)	190
	Beef, Sliced in Gravy (Morton House	1 can (4 1/6 oz)	180
	Chicken A La King (Swanson)	5¼ oz	190
	Stew, Beef (Swanson)	7½ oz	190
	Stew, Lamb (B&M)	1 cup	190
	Chinese Style (Swanson Entree)	8½ oz	200
	Stew, Beef (Van Camp)	1 cup	205
	Chicken & Dumplings (Swanson)	7½ oz	230
R	Turkey w Potatoes (Swanson TV Entree)	8¾ oz	260
	Chile con Carne w Beans (Swanson)	7¾ oz	300
	English Style (Swanson Entree)	5 oz	300
	Chile w Beans (Van Camp	1 cup	315
	Meatballs w Potatoes (Swanson TV Entree)	9 oz	320
	Pot Pie, Beef (Morton	8 oz	370
	Salisbury Steak w Potatoes (Swanson TV Entree)	5½ oz	370
	Chicken, Fried w Potatoes (Swanson TV Entree)	7 oz	380
	Pot Pie, Turkey (Swanson Deep Dish)	½ (8 oz)	380
	Pot Pie, Beef (Swanson Deep Dish)	½ (8 oz)	385
	Pot Pie, Tuna (Morton)	8 oz	385
	Pot Pie, Turkey (Morton)	8 oz	410
	Corned Beef Hash (Van Camp)	1 cup	420
	Pot Pie, Beef (Swanson)	8 oz	445
	Pot Pie, Chicken (Morton)	8 oz	445
	Mexican Style (Swanson Entree)	10 oz	450
	Pot Pie, Turkey (Swanson)	8 oz	450
	Pot Pie, Chicken (Swanson)	8 oz	460

FISH

	Anchovies, Pickled, Canned	1	7
	Clams, Raw, Cherrystone or Little Necks, Meat Only	1	15
	Salmon, Smoked	1 oz	50
	Scallops, Frozen, Breaded	1 oz	50
G	Scallops, Frozen, Breaded	1 (15-20 per lb.)	50
	Crabmeat, Steamed	3 oz	80
	Herring, Canned, Smoked, Kippered	4⅜x1¾x¼"	80
	Lobster, Northern, Cooked	3 oz	80
	Crabmeat, Canned, Drained	3 oz	90
	Rock Fish, Oversteamed	3 oz	90
	Roe, Herring, Canned	3 oz	100
	Shrimp, Canned	3 oz	100
	Bluefish, Baked or Broiled w Butter or Margarine	3 oz	140
	Bluefish, Fried	3 oz	140
	Haddock, Pan-fried or Oven-fried	3 oz	140
	Swordfish, Broiled w Butter or Margarine	3 oz	140
	Halibut, Broiled w Butter or Margarine	3 oz	150
	Clams, Canned, Drained, Chopped or Minced	1 cup	160
	Salmon, Steak, Broiled or Baked w Butter or Margarine	3 oz	160
	Bass, Striped, Oven-fried	3 oz	170
	Flounder, Baked w Butter or Margarine	3 oz	170
	Sardines in Tomato Sauce (Underwood)	can (3¾ oz)	170
	Ocean Perch, Atlantic, Fried	3 oz	190
Y	Shrimp, French-fried	3 oz	190
	Mackerel, Atlantic, Broiled w Butter or Margarine	3 oz	200
	Sardines in Mustard Sauce (Underwood)	can (3¾ oz)	200
	Oysters, Eastern, Raw, Meat Only	1 cup (4-6 med)	220
	Sardines in Oil, Drained (Underwood)	can (3¾ oz)	230
	Tuna in Water	6½ oz	275
	Salmon, Pink, Canned (Del Monte)	7¾ oz	310
	Sardines in Tomator Sauce (Del Monte)	7½ oz	330
	Salmon, Red Sockeye, Canned (Del Monte)	7¾ oz	340
	Tuna, Chunk, Light in Oil (Chicken of Sea)	1 can (6.5 oz)	470

FRESH FRUIT

	Kumquats, Raw with	1 med	12
Y	Lemons, Raw	1 med (2⅛" diam)	20
	Plums, Raw with skin	1 (2⅛" diam)	30

Casaba Melon, Raw	2"x7¾" wedge	40
Peaches, Raw	1 (2½" diam)	40
Tangelo, Raw	1 med (2 1/16" diam)	40
Tangerines, Raw	1 (2⅜" diam)	40
Watermelon, Raw, Diced	1 cup	40
Cherries, Raw, Sweet, Whole	10	45
Cranberries, Raw	1 cup	45
Grapefruit, White Seedless	½ med	45
Grapefruit, Pink, Seedless, Raw	½ med (36" diam)	50
Y Honeydew Melon	7"x2" wedge	50
Papaya, Raw, 4" cubes	1 cup	55
Apricots, Raw with skin	3 (12/lb)	60
Oranges, Raw	1 (2⅜" diam)	60
Strawberries, Raw, Whole, Capped	1 cup	60
Grapes, Raw, American Type	1 cup	70
Peaches, Raw, Sliced	1 cup	70
Raspeberries, Red, Raw	1 cup	70
Apples, Raw with skin	1 med ?3/lb)	80
Blackberries, Raw	1 cup	80
Canteloupe, Raw	½ (5" diam	80
Pineapple, Raw, Diced	1 cup	80
Blueberries, Raw	1 cup	90
Cherries, Raw, Pitted	1 cup	90
Grapefruit, Pink, Raw, Sections	1 C w 2 Tbsp. Juice	90
Grapefruit, White, Raw, Sections	1 C w 2 Tbsp Juice	90
Loganberries, Raw	1 cup	90
Nectarines, Raw with skin	1 (2½" diam)	90
Oranges, Section without membranes	1 cup	90
Bananas, Raw	(1 med 8¾")	100
R Cherries, Raw, Sweet, Pitted	1 cup	100
Pears, Raw with skin	1 (3½" x 2½")	100
Pears, Raw, Sliced with Skin	1 cup	100
Pomegranate, Raw	1 (3⅜"r diam)	100
Raspberries, Black, Raw	1 cup	100
Grapes, Raw, European Type (Adherent Skin)	1 cup	100
Watermelon	1/16 (10"x16" melon)	110
Bananas, Raw, Sliced	1 cup	110
Mango, Raw	1 cup	130
Prunes, "Softenized", Uncooked	10 med	160
Avocado, Raw, California	½	190
Avocado, Raw, Florida, ½" Cubes	1 cup	190
Avocado, Raw Florida	½	200
Prunes, Cooked, Unsweetened	1 cup with liquid	250

Rhubarb, Cooked, Sweetned	1 cup	380
R Raisins, Seedless	1 cup pressed down	480
Dates, Pitted, Chopped	1 cup	480

FROSTINGS

Cherry Fluff (Betty Crocker)	1/12 pkg.	60
Lemon Fluff (Betty Crocker Sunkist)	1/12 pkg.	60
White Fluff (Betty Crocker)	1/12 pgk.	60
Cake & Cookie Decorator, All Colors	1 tbsp.	70
White (Pillsbury Fluffy)	½ pkg.	70
Chocolate Fluff (Betty Crocker)	1/12 pkg.	80
Chocolate Whipped (Betty Crocker)	1/12 pkg.	100
Lemon Whipped (Betty Crocker Sunkist)	1/12 pkg.	100
Strawberry Cream Whipped (Betty Crocker)	1/12 pkg.	100
Vanila Whipped (Betty Crocker)	1/12 pkg.	100
Coconut Pecan (Betty Crocker)	1/12 pkg.	110
Double Dutch, (Pills. Rich 'n Easy)	1/12 pkg.	140
Banana (Betty Crocker Chiquita)	1/12 pkg.	150
Butter Brickle (Betty Crocker)	1/12 pkg.	150
Butter Pecan (Betty Crocker)	1/12 pkg.	150
Caramel Apple (Betty Crocker)	1/12 pkg.	150
Caramel, Golden (Betty Crocker)	1/12 pgk.	150
Cherry, Creamy (Betty Crocker)	1/12 pkg.	150
Cherry Fudge (Betty Crocker)	1/12 pkg.	150
Chocolate, Dark Fudge (Betty Crocker)	1/12 pkg.	150
R Chocolate Fudge (Pillsbury)	1/12 pkg.	150
Chocolate, Light (Pillsbury)	1/12 pkg.	150
Chocolate Malt (Betty Crocker)	1/12 pkg.	150
Chocolate, Milk (Betty Crocker)	1/12 pkg.	150
Chocolate Milk (Pillsbury Rich 'n Easy)	1/12 pkg.	150
Chocolate Walnut (Betty Crocker)	1/12 pkg.	150
Coconut Pecan (Pillsbury's)	1/12 pkg.	150
Coconut Toasted (Betty Crocker)	1/12 pkg.	150
Double Dutch (Pillsbury)	1/12 pkg.	150
Fudge Nugget (Betty Crocker)	1/12 pkg.	150
Lemon (Betty Crocker Sunkist)	1/12 pkg.	150
Lemon (Pillsbury)	1/12 pkg.	150
Orange (Betty Crocker Sunkist)	1/12 pkg.	150
Pineapple (Betty Crocker Dole)	1/12 pkg.	150
Sour Cream Chocolate Fudge (Betty Crocker)	1/12 pkg.	150
Sour Cream White (Betty Crocker)	1/12 pgk.	150
Spice, Creamy (Betty Crocker)	1/12 pkg.	150
Strawberry (Pillsbury Rich 'n Easy)	1/12 pkg.	150
Strawberry, (Pillsbury)	1/12 pkg.	150
Vanilla (Pillsbury)	1/12 pkg.	150
Butter Pecan (Betty Crocker)	1/12 can	160
Caramel (Pillsbury Rich 'n Easy)	1/12 pkg.	160
Cherry, (Betty Crocker)	1/12 can	160
Chocolate Fudge (Betty Crocker)	1/12 pkg.	160

Chocolate Fudge (Pillsbury Rich 'n Easy).................................1/12 pkg. 160
Chocolate Milk (Betty Crocker)...................................1/12 can 160
Chocolate Nut (Betty Crocker)...................................1/12 can 160
Dark Dutch (Betty Crocker)...................1/12 can 160
Lemon (Betty Crocker sunkist ....1/12 can 160
R Orange, (Betty Crocker Sunkist)............1/12 can 160
Sour Cream White (Betty Crocker) ....1/12 can 160
Vanilla, (Pillsbury Rich 'n Easy) ....1/12 pkg. 160
White, Creamy (Betty Crocker)...............1/12 can 160
Chocolate (Betty Crocker)........................1/12 can 170
Coconut Almond (Pillsbury)...................1/12 pg. 170
prep.
Sour Cream Chocolate (Betty Crocker) ....1/12 can 170

FROZEN DINNERS

Beef (Morton)	11 oz	295
Macaroni & Cheese (Morton)..................	12¾ oz.	315
Spaghetti & Meat Balls (Morton)............	12½ oz.	320
Macaron & Beef (Morton)	11 oz.	370
Spaghetti & Meat Balls (Morton)............	11 oz	370
Chicken & Dumplings (Morton)................	12 oz.	370
Beef (Swanson TV)................................	11½ oz.	370
Fish (Morton)......................................	8¾ oz.	375
Noodles & Chicken (Swanson TV)	10¼ oz.	380
Shrimp (Morton)..................................	7¾ oz.	380
Swiss Steak (Swanson TV)......................	10 oz.	380
Ham (Swanson TV)	10¼ oz.	380
Salisbury Steak (Morton........................	11 oz.	385
Meat Loaf (Morton)..............................	11 oz.	400
Macaroni & Beef (Swanson TV)..............	12 oz.	410
Ham (Morton)......................................	10 z.	430
Filet of Ocean Fish (Swanson TV)	11½ oz.	440
Fish n Chips (Swanson TV)......................	10¼ oz.	450
Turkey (Morton)	12 oz.	450
Chicken, Fried (Morton)........................	11 oz.	480
Salisbury Steak (Swanson TV)	11½ oz.	500
R Polynesian Style (Swanson)	12¼ oz.	510
Salisbury Steak (Swanson) 3-Course)..	16 oz.	510
Italian Style (Swanson)........................	13½ oz.	510
Veal Parmigiana (Swanson TV)	12¼ oz.	520
Meat Loaf (Swason 3-Course)	16½ oz.	540
Beef (Swanson 3-Course)......................	15 oz.	540
Turkey (Swanson 3-Course)...................	16 oz.	550
Beans and Franks (Swanson TV)	11¼ oz.	550
Beans and Frankfurters (Morton)...........	12 oz.	560
Beef (Morton 3-Course)........................	17 oz.	565
Enchilada, Beef (Swanson TV)	15 oz.	570
Chicken, Fried (Swanson TV)..................	11½ oz.	570
Salisbury Steak (Morton 3-Course)..	17 oz.	610
Mexican Style (Swanson 3-Course)..	18 oz.	620
Turkey (Morton 3-Course).....................	17 oz.	635
Meat Loaf (Morton 3-Course).................	17 oz.	650
Chicken, Fried (Swanson 3-Course)..	15 oz.	670
Turkey, (Swanson Hungry Man)............	15 oz.	670
Mexican Style (Swanson)	19 oz.	690
Chicken & Dumplings (Morton 3-Course)...............................	16½ oz.	770
R Chicken, Bonelss (Swanson Hungry Man).....................................	19 oz.	770
Chicken, Fried (Morton 3-Course)...........	17 oz.	870
Salisbury Steak (Swanson Hungry Man).....................................	17 oz.	930
Chicken, Fried (Swanson Hungry Man).....................................	15¾ oz	960

FRUIT—CANNED AND FROZEN

Grapefruit, Sections, Canned in Juice (Del Monte)........................	1 cup	90
Mandarin Oranges, Canned (Del Monte)	5 oz	90
Cherries Canned, Red Sour (Stokely-Van Camp).........................	1 cup	100
Mixed, Canned (Del Monte Fruit Cup)..	5 oz	100
Peaches, Canned, Spiced (Del Monte)	5 oz	100
Peaches, Canned, Cling, Diced (Del Monte Fruit Cup)	5 oz	110
Grapefruit, Sections, Canned in Syrup (Del Monte)	1 cup	140
Pineapple, Canned in Juice (Del Monte)	1 cup	140
Pineapple, Canned in Juice Chunk or Crushed (Libby's)..................	1 cup	140
Pinneapple, Canned in Juice, Sliced (Libby's)................................	4 sl	140
Pears, canned (Del Monte Bartlett).........	1 cup	160
Grapefruit, Sections, Canned (Stokley-Van Camp)........................	1 cup	160
R Applesauce (Del Monte)......................	1 cup	170
Fruit Cocktail, Canned (Del Monte)..........	1 cup	170
Fruits for Salad, Canned (Del Monte).....	1 cup	170
Peaches, Canned (Stokely-Van Camp)...	1 cup	170
Peaches, Canned, Freestone (Del Monte)	1 cup	170
Pineapple, Canned (Stokely-Van Camp)...	1 cup	170
Rhubarb, Frozen (Bird's Eye)..................	1 cup	170
Fruit Cocktail, Canned (Stokely Van Camp)....................................	1 cup	175
Cherries, Canned, Dark, Sweetened in Pits (Del Monte)	1 cup	180
Fruits for Salad, Canned (Libby's)..........	1 cup	180
Peaches, Canned (Stokely-Van Camp)..	1 cup	180
Peaches, Frozen, Sliced (Bird's Eye)..	1 cup	180
Pears, Canned (Stokely-Van Camp)........	1 cup	180
Cherries, Canned, Dark, Sweetened, Pitted (Del Monte)	1 cup	190
Cherries, Canned, Light, Sweetened w pits (Del Monte)	1 cup	190
Peaches, Canned, Cling, Sliced (Libby's)..	1 cup	190
Pears, Canned (Libby's)	1 cup	190
Pineapple, Canned in Syrup (Del Monte)	1 cup	190

206   (G)=Green   (Y)=Yellow   (R)=Red

Pineapple, Canned, in Heavy Syrup, Sliced (Libby's)	1 cup	190
Plums, Canned, Purple (Del Monte)	1 cup	190
Apricots, Canned, Whole (Del Monte)	1 cup	200
Apricots, Canned Halves (Del Monte)	1 cup	200
Apricots, Canned (Libby's)	1 cup	200
Cherries, Canned, Dark and Sweet (Stokely-Van Camp)	1 cup	200
Cherries, Canned, Light (Stokely-Van Camp)	1 cup	200
Figs in Heavy Syrup (Stokely-Van Camp)	1 cup	200
Fruit Coctail, Canned (Libby's)	1 cup	200
Fruit Salad, Canned (Del Monte)	1 cup	200
Plums, Canned (Stokely-Van Camp)	1 cup	200
R Strawberries, Frozen Whole (Bird's Eye)	½ pkg.	200
Apricots Canned (Stokely-Van Camp)	1 cup	210
Figs, Canned (Del Monte)	1 cup	210
Mixed, Frozen (Bird's Eye Quick Thaw)	1 cup	220
Applesauce, Canned (Stokely-Van Camp)	1 cup	220
Blueberries, Frozen (Bird's Eye Quick Thaw)	1 cup	230
Prunes, Canned, Stewed (Del Monte)	1 cup	230
Fruit Cocktail, Canned (S&W)	1 cup	240
Cherries, Frozen (Bird's Eye Quick Thaw)	1 cup	245
Peaches, Canned, Cling, Sliced (Libby's)	1 cup	250
Strawberries, Frozen (Bird's Eye Quick Thaw)	1 cup	250
Raspberries, Frozen (Bird's Eye Quick Thaw)	1 cup	300
Strawberries, Frozen, Halves (Bird's Eye)	1 cup	325

FRUIT-DRINKS

Cranberry-Apple (Ocean Spray Cranapple Low Cal)	6 fl. oz.	30
Cranberry Juice Cocktail (Ocean Spray Low Cal)	6 fl. oz.	40
Gatorade	6 fl. oz.	55
Lemonade (Funny Face)	6 fl. oz.	60
Raspberry (Funny Face)	6 fl. oz.	60
Strawberry (Funny Face)	6 fl. oz.	60
Tutti Frutti (Funny Face)	6 fl. oz.	60
Watermelon (Funny Face)	6 fl. oz.	60
R Cherry (Funny Face)	6 fl. oz.	70
Grape (Funny Face)	6 fl. oz.	70
Grapefruit, Canned, Unsweetened (Del Monte)	6 fl. oz.	70
Lemonade, Frozen, Reconstituted (Minute Maid)	6 fl. oz.	75
Lemonade, Frozen, Reconstituted (Snow Crop)	6 fl. oz.	75
Lemon-Limeade, Frozen, Reconstituted (Min. Maid)	6 fl. oz.	75
Lemon-Limeade, Frozen, Reconstituted (Snow Crop)	6 fl. oz.	75

Limeade, Frozen, Reconstituted (Minute Maid)	6 fl. oz.	75
Limeade, (Snow Crop)	6 fl. oz.	75
Grapefruit, Canned, Sweetned (Del Monte)	6 fl. oz.	80
Cherry (Lipton)	6 fl. oz.	85
Grape (Lipton)	6 fl. oz.	85
Lemon (Lipton)	6 fl. oz.	85
Orange (Lipton)	6 fl. oz.	85
Punch (Lipton)	6 fl. oz.	85
Apple (Hi-C)	6 fl. oz.	90
Cherry (Hi-C)	6 fl. oz.	90
Citrus Cooler (Hi-C)	6 fl. oz.	90
Grape (Tang)	6 fl. oz.	90
Grape (Welchade)	6 fl. oz.	90
Grape, Red (Welchade)	6 fl. oz.	90
Grape, White (Welchade)	6 fl. oz.	90
Grapefruit (Tang)	6 fl. oz.	90
Orange (Start)	6 fl. oz.	90
Orange (Tang)	6 fl. oz.	90
Orange (Welchade)	6 fl. oz.	90
Orange (Welch's Sunshake Breakfast Drink)	6 fl. oz.	90
peneapple-Grapefruit, Canned (Del Monte)	6 fl. oz.	90
R Pineapple-Orange, Canned (Del Monte)	6 fl. oz.	90
Pineapple-Pink, Grapefruit, Canned (Del Monte)	6 fl. oz.	90
Punch, Apple, Red (Hawaiian Punch)	6 fl. oz.	90
Wild Berry (Hi-C)	6 fl. oz.	90
Orangeade, Frozen, Reconstit. Minute Maid)	6 fl. oz.	95
Orangeade, Frozen, Reconstit. (Snow Crop)	6 fl. oz.	95
Peach (Alegre Paradise Peach)	6 fl. oz.	96
Grape (Hi-C)	6 fl. oz.	100
Orange (Hi-C)	6 fl. oz.	100
Orange-Pineapple (Hi-C)	6 fl. oz.	100
Punch, Florida (Hi-C)	6 fl. oz.	100
Punch, Tropical Fruit (Alegre)	6 fl. oz.	100
Strawberry Cooler (Hi-C)	6 fl. oz.	100
Cranberry Juice Cocktail (Welch's)	6 fl. oz.	105
Grape (Welch's sunshake Breakfast Drink)	6 fl. oz.	105
Orange (Alegre)	6 fl. oz.	105
Cranberry Juice Cocktail (Ocean Spray)	6 fl. oz.	110
Cranberry Juice, Frozen, Recon. (Welch's)	6 fl. oz.	110
Cranberry-Apple (Welche's)	6 fl. oz.	120
Punch, Fruit Juicy Red (Hawaiian Punch)	6 fl. oz.	120
Punch, Great Grape (Hawaiian Punch)	6 fl. oz.	120
Punch, Very Berry (Hawaiian Punch)	6 fl. oz.	120
Mango-Pineapple (Alegre'	6 fl. oz.	140

FRUIT JUICES

Y Lemon Frozen, Ronst. (Minute Maid)	6 fl. oz.	40

(G)=Green (Y)=Yellow (R)=Red 207

Lemon Frozen, Reconst. (Snow Crop)	6 fl. oz.	40
Lemon, Fresh	6 fl. oz.	45
Lime, Fresh	6 fl. oz.	45
Grapefruit, Canned, Unsweetened (Del Monte)	6 fl. oz.	70
Orange, Canned, Sweetened (Del Monte)	6 fl. oz.	70
Grapefruit, Fresh	6 fl. oz.	75
Y Grapefruit, Frozen Reconst. (Minute Maid)	6 fl. oz.	75
Grapefruit, Frozen, Reconst. (Snow Crop)	6 fl. oz.	75
Orange, Frozen, Reconst. (Bird's Eye)	6 fl. oz.	75
Orange-Grapefruit, Frozen Reconst. (Min. Maid)	6 fl. oz.	75
Orange-Grapefruit Frozen, Reconst. (Snow Crop)	6 fl. oz.	75
Grapefruit, Canned, Sweetened (Del Monte)	6 fl. oz.	80
Orange-Grapefruit Canned, Sweetened (Del Monte)	6 fl. oz.	80
Orange-Grapefruit, Canned, Unsweetened (Del Monte)	6 fl. oz.	80
Grapefruit, Canned, Unsweetened (Stokely VC)	6 fl. oz.	85
Orange—Fresh	6 fl. oz.	85
Orange, Dairy Case (Min. Maid)	6 fl. oz.	85
Orange, Imitation, Frozen Recost. (Awake)	6 fl. oz.	85
Tangerine, Frozen, Reconst. (Min. Maid)	6 fl. oz.	85
Tangarine, Frozen, Reconst. (Snow Crop)	6 fl. oz.	85
Orange, Canned, Unsweetened (Stokely VC)	6 fl. oz.	90
Orange, Frozen, Reconst. (Min. Maid)	6 fl. oz.	90
Orange, Frozen, Reconst. (Snow Crop)	6 fl. oz.	90
Apricot Nectar (Del Monte)	6 fl. oz.	100
R Grape, Frozen, Reconst. (Min. Maid)	6 fl. oz.	100
Grape, Frozen, Reconst. (Snow Crop)	6 fl. oz.	100
Grape, Frozen, Reconst. (Welch's)	6 fl. oz.	100
Grapefruit, Canned Sweetened (Stokely VC)	6 fl. oz.	100
Orange, Canned, Sweetened (Stokely VC)	6 fl. oz.	100
Orange, Imitation (Bright Early)	6 fl. oz.	100
Orange, Imitation Frozen, Reconst. (Orange Plus)	6 fl. oz.	100
Orange-Grapefruit, Canned, Sweetened (Stokely)	6 fl. oz.	100
Peach Nectar, Canned (Del Monte)	6 fl. oz.	100
Pineapple, Canned (Del Monte)	6 fl. oz.	100
Pineapple, Canned Unsweetened (Libby's)	6 fl. oz.	100
Pineapple, Canned Unsweetened (Stikely)	6 fl. oz.	100
Grape, Red, Frozen, Reconst. (Welch's)	6 fl. oz.	110

Pear Nectar, Canned (Del Monte)	6 fl. oz.	110
Grape, Bottled (Welch's)	6 fl. oz.	120
R Grape, White, Frozen, Reconst. (Welch's)	6 fl. oz.	120
Prune, Canned (Del Monte)	6 fl. oz.	120

GELATIN

All Regular Flavors (Jell-O)	½ cup	80
Y All Wild Flavors (Jell-O)	½ cup	80
All Flavors (Jell-O 1-2-3)	½ cup	90

ICE CREAM & ICE MILK

Ice bar (Kool Pops)	1 bar	27
Y Iced milk bar (Eskimo Rainbow)	1 bar	68
Weight Watcher's Snack Cup	1 cup (5 oz)	100
Hardened Ice milk	1 cup	200
Flavored Ice water	1 cup	250
R Ice cream (10% fat)	1 cup	260
Ice milk (soft serve)	1 cup	270
Ice cream (soft serve)	1 cup	330

LEGUMES

Cowpeas, (Black-Eye) Dr, Cooked, Drained	1 cup	190
Beans, Great Northern, Dry Cooked, Drained	1 cup	210
Lentils Dry, Cooked	1 cup	210
Beans, Navy, Pea, Dry, Cooked, Drained	1 cup	220
Beans, Red Kidney, Dry, Cooked, Drained	1 cup	220
Beans, Baked-Style, Vegetarian (Heinz)	1 can (8 oz)	230
Peas, Split, Dry, Cooked	1 cup	230
Beans, Baked-Style w Pork (Heinz)	½ can	250
Beans, Baked-Style w Pork (Campbell's)	8 oz.	260
R Beans, Lima, Dry, Cooked, Drained	1 cup	260
Beans, Baked-Style (Campbell's Barbecue)	8 oz.	280
Beans, Baked-Style (van Camps)	1 cup	280
Beans, Baked-Style w Beef (Campbell's)	7½ oz.	280
Beans, Baked-Style (Campbell's Old Fashioned)	8 oz.	290
Beans, Baked-Style w Pork (Campbell's Home Style)	1 cup	300
Beans, Baked-Style w Frankfurters (Van Camp's Beanne & Weenie)	1 cup	340
Beans, Baked (B&M)	1 cup	340
Beans, Baked, Red Kidney Homemaker's	1 cup	340
Beans, Baked, Red Kidney (B&M)	1 cup	360
Beans, Baked, Yellow Eye (B&M)	1 cup	360
Beans, Baked-style w Frankfurters (Campbell's)	8 oz.	370

208   (G)=Green   (Y)=Yellow   (R)=Red

MEAT

Item	Amount	Calories
Smokies, Little (Oscar Mayer)	1	30
Vienna Sausage, Canned (Van Camp)	1	35
Frankfurters (Oscar Mayer Little Wieners)	1	35
Vienna Sausage, Canned (Oscar Mayer)	1	45
Saussage, New England Brand (Oscar Mayer)	2 sl.	60
Ham, Sliced, Smoked, Cooked (Oscar Mayer)	2 sl.	60
Gourmet Loaf (Ekrich)	2 sl.	60
Salami, Hard (Oscar Mayer)	2 sl.	80
Gourmet Loaf (Ekrich)	2 sl.	80
Honey Loaf (Oscar Mayer)	2 sl.	80
Bacon, Cooked (Oscar Mayer)	2 sl.	80
Smokettes, Beef	1	85
Smok-y Links (Ekrich)	1	85
Bacon, Canadian (Oscar Mayer)	2 sl.	90
Corned Beef Loaf (Oscar Mayer)	2 sl.	90
Honey Style Loaf (Ekrich)	2 sl.	90
Salami, Beef Cotto (Oscar Mayer)	2 sl.	100
Salami, Cotto (Oscar Mayer)	2 sl.	100
Salami for Beer (Oscar Mayer)	2 sl.	100
Bar-B-Q Loaf (Oscar Mayer)	2 sl.	100
Ham, Canned (Oscar Mayer Jubilee)	3 oz.	105
Banquet Loaf (Ekrich Beef Smorgas Pac)	2 sl.	110
Salami, Beef, Machiach Brand (Oscar Mayer)	2 sl.	120
Y Ham, Sliced, Boneless (Oscar Mayer Jubilee)	3 oz.	120
Smokie Links (Oscar Mayer)	1	130
Ham, Chopped (Oscar Mayer)	2 sl.	130
Old Fashioned Loaf (Oscar Mayer)	2 sl.	130
Olive Loaf (Oscar Mayer)	2 sl.	130
Pickle & Pimento Loaf (Oscar Mayer)	2 sl.	130
Picnic Loaf (Oscar Mayer)	2 sl.	130
Beef Pickle Loaf (Ekrich Beef Smorgas Pac)	2 sl.	130
Summer Sausage (Beef Oscar Mayer)	2 ls.	140
Bologna, Beef (Oscar Mayer)	2 sl.	140
Bologna (Oscar Mayer)	2 sl.	140
Frankfurters (Oscar Mayer Wieners)	1	140
Frankfurters, Beef (Oscar Mayer)	1	140
Ham Steak (Oscar Mayer Jubilee)	2 sl.	140
Ham & Cheese Loaf (Oscar Mayer)	2 sl.	140
Summer Sausage (Oscar Mayer)	2 sl.	150
Ham, Canned (Oscar Mayer Omca)	3 oz.	150
Old Fashioned Loaf (Ekrich)	2 sl.	150
Frankfurter's, Beef (Ekrich Fun Franks)	1	155
Skinless Franks (Ekrich Fun Franks)	1	155
Smokies, (Ekrich) 1 lb. pkg.	1	160
Beef, Chuck, Braised, Simmered or Pot Roast Lean & Fat	3 oz.	160
Bologna, Thick Sliced (Ekrich) 12 oz. pkg.	1 sl.	160
Bologna, Beef (Eckrich)	2 sl.	160
Beef Steak, Round, Braised, Broiled or Sauteed, Lean only	3 oz.	160
Ham, Cured, Roasted, Lean Only	3 oz.	160
Lamb, Leg, Roasted, Lean Only	3 oz.	160
Lamb, Leg, Roasted, Lean Only	3 oz.	160
Heart, Beef, Braised, Lean	3 oz.	160
Smokies (Eckrich), 12 oz. pkg.	1	165
Bologna, Thick Sliced (Eckrich) 1 lb. pkg.	1 sl.	170
Beef Steak, Flank, cooked	3 oz.	170
Beef Plate, Simmered, Lean Only	3 oz.	170
Pickle Loaf (Eckrich)	2 sl.	170
Lamb, Shoulder, Roasted, Lean Only	3 oz.	170
Veal Cutlets, Braised or Broiled, Medium Fat	3 oz.	180
Y Bologna (Ekrich Sandwich)	2 sl.	180
Beef Steak, Sirloin, Broiled, Lean Only	3 oz.	180
Beef, Roast, Rump, Cooked, Lean Only	3 oz.	180
Beef, Dried or Chipped	3 oz.	180
Braunschweiger Liver Sausage, Sliced (Oscar Mayer)	2 sl.	180
Frankfurters, Beef Machiach Brand (Oscar Mayer)	1	180
Ham, Fresh, Roasted, Lean Only	3 oz.	180
Lamb Chop, Rib, Cooked Only	3 oz.	180
Bologna, Sliced (Eckrich)	2 sl.	190
Bologna, Beef (Eckrich) 12 oz. pkg.	2 sl.	190
Beef Steak, Club, Porterhouse or T-Bone, Broiled, Lean Only	3 oz.	190
Beef, Gound, Broiled Well-Don, Lean	3 oz.	190
Frankfurters (Eckrich Jumbo Fun Franks)	1	190
Kielbasa, Links (Ekrich Polska)	1	190
Sandwich Spread (Oscar Mayer)	3 oz.	195
Veal, Boneless Custs, Braised, Pot Roasted or Stewed, Medium Fat	3 oz.	200
Veal, Loin, Braised, or Broiled, Med. Fat	3 oz.	200
Luncheon Meat (Oscay Mayer)	2 sl.	200
Liver, Beef, Fried	3 oz.	200
Tongue, Beef, Braised Medium Fat	3 oz.	210
Beef Roast, Rib, Cooked, Lean Only	3 oz.	210
Ham, Cured, Roasted, Gound, Lean Only	1 cup	210
R Liver, Hog, Fried	3 oz.	210.
Kidney, Beef, Braised	3 oz.	210
Pork, Cured, Boston Butt or Picnic, Roasted, Lean Only	3 oz.	210
Pork, shoulder, Roasted, Lean Only	3 oz.	210
Liver Cheese (Oscar Mayer)	3 oz.	210
Beef Steak, Round, Braised, Broiled or Sauteed, Lean & Fat	3 oz.	220
Liver, Calf, Fried	3 oz.	220
Pork, Loin, Baked or Roasted, Lean Only	3 oz.	220
Pork Chop, Loin, Broiled, Lean Only	3 oz.	225

Food	Amount	Calories
Veal, Rib, Roasted	3 oz.	230
Beef Roast, Rump, Cooked, Ground, Lean Only	1 cup	230
Ham, Fresh, Roasted, Gound Lean Only	1 cup	240
Lamb, Leg, Roasted, Lean & Fat	3 oz.	250
Beef, Chuck, Braised, Simmered or Pot Roasted, Lean	3 oz.	250
Ham, Cured, Roasted, Lean	3 oz.	250
Corned Beef Spread (Underwood) (4½ oz.)	1 can	250
Ham, Cured, Roasted, Diced, Lean Only	1 cup	260
Lamb, Leg, Roasted, Diced, Lean Only	1 cup	260
Beef, Chuck, Cooked, Diced, Lean Only	1 cup	270
Beef, Gound, Broiled Well-Done, Regular	3 oz.	270
Heart, Beef, Braised, Diced, Lean	1 cup	270
Pork, Cured, Boston Butt or Picnic Roasted, Ground Lean Only	1 cup	270
Pork Shoulder, Roasted, Gound, Lean Only	1 cup	270
Sweetbreads, Beef, Braised	3 oz.	270
Port, Cured, Boston Butt or Picnic	3 oz.	285
Roasted Lean Fat	3 oz.	285
Sausage, Smoked, Skinless (Eckrich)	3 oz.	285
Bologna, Garlic Ring (Eckrich)	3 oz.	285
Bologna, Lunch (Eckrich)	3 oz.	285
Bologna, Pickled Ring (Echrich)	3 oz.	285
Bologna, Ring (Eckrich)	3 oz.	285
R Luncheon Meat, Canned (Oscar Mayer)	3 oz.	285
Port Luncheon Meat, Canned (Oscar Mayer)	3 oz.	285
Beef Roast, Rump, Cooked, Diced Lean Only	1 cup	290
Lamb, Shoulder, Roasted, Lean & Fat **Y**	3 oz.	290
Lamb, Shoulder, Roasted, Diced, Lean Only	1 cup	290
Veal, Rib, Roasted, Ground	1 cup	300
Beef Roast, Rump Cooked, Lean & Fat **R**	3 oz.	300
Braunschweiger (Oscar Mayer)	3 oz.	300
Ham, Fresh, Roasted, Diced, Lean Only	1 cup	300
Lamb Chop, Loin, Cooked, Lean Only	1 cup	300
Kielbasa (Eckrich Polska)	3 oz.	300
Pork Shoulder, Roasted, Lean & Fat	3 oz.	300
Pork, Loin, Baked or Roasted, Lean & Fat	3 oz.	310
Sausage, Smoked (Eckrich H.C.)	3 oz.	315
Corned Beef, Fresh, Cooked	3 oz.	320
Ham, Fresh, Roasted, Lean & Fat **R**	3 oz.	320
Pork Chop, Loin, Broiled. Lean & Fat	3 oz.	320
Veal, Boneless Cuts, Braised, Pot Roasted or Stewed, Med. Fat, chopped	1 cup	330
Veal, Loin, Braised or Broiled. Diced Med. Fat	1 cup	330
Beef Steak, Sirloin, Broiled, Lean & Fat	3 oz.	330
Pork, Cured, Boston Butt or Picnic, Roasted, Diced, Lean Only	1 cup	340
Pork, Shoulder, Roasted, Diced, Lean Only	1 cup	340
Lamb Chop, Rib, Cooked, Lean & Fat	3 oz.	360
Pork, Loin, Baked or Roasted, Diced, Lean Only	1 cup	360
Spareribs, Braised, Lean & Fat	3 oz.	370
Beef Plate, Simmered, Lean & Fat	3 oz.	370
Beef Roast, Rib, Cooked, Lean & Fat	3 oz.	370
Veal, Rib, Roasted, Diced	1 cup	380
Ham & Cheese Spread (Spreadables)	1 can	400
R Beef Steak, Club, Porterhouse or T-Bone, Boiled, Lean & Fat	3 oz.	400
Beef, Chuck, Cooked, Diced, Lean & Fat	1 cup	410
Ham, Cured, Roasted, Diced, Lean & Fat	1 cup	410
Ham, Deviled, Canned (Underwood) (4¾ oz.)	1 can	440
Ham Salad (Spreadables)	1 can	450
Lamb, shoulder, Roasted, Diced, Lean & Fat	1 cup	470
Beef Roast, Rump, Cooked, Diced, Lean & Fat	1 cup	490
corned Beef Spread (Spreadables)	1 can	500
Pork, Baked or Roasted, Diced, Lean & Fat	1 cup	510
Ham, Fresh, Roasted, Diced, Lean & Fat	1 cup	520

MILK

Food	Amount	Calories
Milk, Dry, Nonfat, Recon-stituted (Carnation) **Y**	1 c	80
Buttermilk, Made from Skim Milk	1 c	90
Milk, Nonfat (Skim)	1 c	90
Milk, Partly Skimmed (2% Fat), Nonfat Milk Solids Added	1 c	150
Milk, Whole, 3.5% Fat **R**	1 c	160
Evaporated Milk, Skimmed (Carnation)	1 c	190
Evaporated Milk (Carnation)	1 c	350

MILK-BEVERAGES

Food	Amount	Calories
Butterscotch, Canned (Carnation Slender)	1 can	225
Chocolate, Canned (Carnation Slender)	1 can	225
Chocolate Fudge, Cenned (Carnation Slender)	1 can	225
R Chocolate Malt, Canned (Carnation Slender)	1 can	225
Chocolate Marshamallow, Canned (Carnation Slender)	1 can	225
Coffee, Canned (Carnation Slender)	1 can	225
Egg Nog, Canned (Carnation Slender)	1 can	225
Vanilla, Canned (Carnation Slender)	1 can	225

Chocolate Malt (Pillsbury Instant Breakfast)	1 pouch w milk	280
Strawberry (Pillsbury Instant Breakfast)	8 fl. oz.	280
Vanilla (Pillsbury Instant Breakfast)	1 pouch w milk	280
Butterscotch, Made w Whole Milk Carnation Instant Bkfst)	8 oz.	290
Chocolate (Pillsbury Instant Breakfast)	1 pouch w milk	280
Chocolate, Made w Whole Milk (Carnation Instant Bkfst)	8 fl. oz.	290
Chocolate Fudge, Made w Whole Milk (Carnation Instant Bkfst)	8 fl. oz.	290
R Chocolate Malt, Made w Whole Milk (Carnation Instant Bkfst)	8 fl. oz.	290
Chocolate Marshmallow. Made w Whole Milk (Carn. Inst. Bkfst)	8 fl. oz.	290
Coffee, Madw w Whole Milk (Carn. Inst. Bkfst.)	8 fl. oz.	290
Egg Nog, Made w Whole Milk (Carn. Inst. Bkfst)	8 fl. oz.	290
Strawberry, Made w Whole Milk (Carn. Inst. Bkfst)	8 fl. oz.	290
Vanilla, Made w Whole Milk (Carn. Inst. Bkfst)	8 fl. oz.	290
Chocolate, Made w Whole Milk (Carn. Special Inst. Bkfst)	8 fl. oz.	350
Strawberry, Made w Whole Milk (Carn. Spec. Inst Bkfst)	8 fl. oz.	350
Vanilla, Made w Whole Milk (Carn. Spec. Inst. Bkfst)	8 fl. oz.	350

MUFFINS

Blueberry (Morton)	1	75
Blueberry (Duncan Hines)	1	90
English (Morton)	1	100
Blueberry (Thomas Toast-r-Cakes)	1	110
Bran (Thomas Toast-r-Cakes)	1	115
Cinnamon-Raisin (Thomas Toast-r-Cakes)	1	115
Corn (Thomas Toast-r-Cakes)	1	115
Strawberry (Thomas Toast-r-Cakes)	1	115
Corn (Dromedary)	1	130
R English, Fresh or Frozen (Thomas)	1	135
English (Wonder)	1	140
English, Onion, Fresh or Frozen (Thomas)	1	140
Scones (Wonder)	1	140
Raisin (Wonder Round)	1	150
Bran with Raisins (Thomas), Small	1	160
Blueberry (Morton Round)	1	170
Cinnamon-Apple (Morton Round)	1	170
Corn (Morton)	1	170
Raisin Bran (Morton Round)	1	170
Corn (Morton Round)	1	175
Corn (Thomas), Small	1	180
Bran with Raisins (Thomas), Large	1	210
Corn, (Thomas), Large	1	235

NUTS & SEEDS

Almonds, in Shell	10	60
Peanuts, Roasted in Shell, Jumbo	10	110
Cashews, Dry Roasted (Skippy)	1 oz	165
Peanuts, Dry Roasted (Skippy)	1 oz	165
Mixed Nuts, Dry Roasted (Skippy)	1 oz.	170
Chestnuts, Fresh, Shelled	1 c	310
Almonds, Shelled, Sliced	1 c	570
Walnuts, English, Halves	1 c (about 50)	650
R Pecans, Halves	1 c	740
Pumpkin Seeds, Dry, Hulled	1 c	770
Squash Seeds, Dry, Hulled	1 c	770
Walnuts, English, Pieces of Chips	1 c	780
Walnuts, Black, Chopped, or Broken Kernels	1 c	790
Sunflower Seeds, Dry, Hulled	1 c	810
Peanuts, Salted, Whole or Halves	1 c	840
Almonds, Shelled, Whole	1 c	850
Filberts, Shelled, Whole Kernels	1 c	860
Brazil Nuts, Shelled	1 c	920

PANCAKES AND WAFFLES (about 32)

Corn Sticks, Frozen (Aunt Jemima)	1	50
Pancake-Waffle (Aunt Jemima Complete)	1 (4″ cake)	55
Waffles, Frozen (Downy Flake Regular)	1	55
Waffles, Frozen (Aunt Jemima Original)	1	60
Waffles, Forzen, Buttermilk (Aunt Jemima)	1 section	60
Pancake-Waffle Mix (Aunt Jemima Original)	1 (4″ cake)	65
Pancake-Waffle Mix, Buckwehat (Aunt Jemima)	1 (4″ cake	65
Pancake Mix (Hungry Jack Complete	1 (4″ cake)	65
R Pancake Mix (Hungry Jack Extra Light)	1 (4″ cake)	75
Pancake-Waffle Mix (Aunt Jemima Complete)	1 (4″ cake)	55
Pancake-Waffle Mix, Buckwheat (Aunt Jemima)	1 (4″ cake)	65
Pancake Mix, Buttermilk (Hungry Jack Complete)	1 (4″ cake)	75
Pancake Mix, Buttermilk (Hungry Jack)	1 (4″ cake)	80
Waffles, Frozen (Downyflake Homade Size)	1	80
Waffles, Frozen, Buttermilk Round (Downyflake)	1	100
Pancake Mix, Buttermilk Duncan Hines)	1 (4″ diam)	110

French Toast, Frozen (Bel-Air)...............1 sl.   115

Pancake Mix, Blueberry

R (Hungry Jack) 1   120

                        (4" cake)

Breakfast Squares

PASTA & PASTA DISHES

Artichoke Imitation Fettuccomo (De Boles)..7 oz.		56
Y	Artichoke Imitation Macaroni (De Boles)..7 oz.	56
Artichoke Imitation Macaroni (San Martin)...7 oz.		56
Artichoke Imitation Spaghetti (De Boles)..7 oz		56
Spaghetti w Tomato Sauce and Cheese canned (Heinz) ....1 can 7½		160
Spaghetti, in Tomato Sauce Canned (Van Camp)....................................1 cup		170
Spaghetti in Tomato Cheese Sauce Canned (Franco American Spathetti-O's).....................................7½ oz		170
Spaghetti w Tomato Sauce and Cheese (Franco-American) ....7½ oz.		180
Macaroni Dry (Golden Grain) ....2 oz		200
Macaroni & Cheese Canned (Franco-American)...............................7¼ oz		200
Noodles, Dry (Golden Grain) ....2 oz		200
Spaghetti Dry (Golden Grain) ....2 oz . 200		
Macaroni, Dry (Buitoni Pasta Romana)..2 oz.		210
Macaroni, High Protein, Dry (Buitoni) ....2 oz.		210
Macaroni & Cheese Canned (Heinz) ....1 can 7½ oz.		210
Spaghetti, Dry (Buitoni Pasta Romana) ....2 oz.		210
Spaghetti, High Protein, Dry (Buitoni) ....2 oz.		210
Macaroni & Beef, Canned (Franco-American)...............................7½ oz.		220
Spagehtti w Meat Balls, Canned (Franco-American)...............................7¼ oz.		230
R	Spaghetti w Meat Balls, Canned (Franco-American Spaghetti-O)...........7½ oz.	230
Spaghetti w Meat Balls Canned (Van Camp) ....1 cup		230
Macaroni & Cheese Mix (Kraft Deluxe Dinner) ....14 oz. box 240 ¾ c prep.		
Ravioli, Beef, Canned (Franco American)..7½ oz.		240
Spaghetti w Beef and Tomato Sauce Canned (Franco-American)...................7½ oz.		250
Noodles and Cheese, Mix (Kraft Dinner)......................................6¼ oz box 255 ¾ c prep.		
Ravioli Beef Frozen (Celeste).................7		260
Spaghetti w Franks Canned (Franco-American Spagehtti-O's) ....7½ oz		260
Spaghetti Dinner Mix (Kraft American Style)....................................8 oz box 260 1 c prep		
Spaghetti Dinner Mix (Kraft Tangy Italian Style) ....8 oz bos 260 1 c prep		
Ravioli, Cheese, Frozen (Celeste) 7		265

Noodles and Beef Sauce (Pennsylvania Dutch Brand)................1 c		275
Italian Style entree, Frozen (Swanson)..9½ oz.		280
Macaroni and Cheese, Mix (Kraft Dinner)......................................7¼ oz box 280 ¾ c prep		
Macaroni & Cheese Mix (Kraft Dinner)......................................14 oz. box 280 ¼ c prep.		
Macaroni & Onion Sauce (Penn. Dutch Brand)..........................1 cup		285
Noodles & Chicken Sauce (Penn Dutch Brand)..........................1 cup		285
Spaghetti and Meat, Frozen (Morton) ....8 oz		290
R	Noodles & Cheese Sauce (Penn. Dutch Brand)..........................1 cup	295
Spaghetti and Cheese, Frozen (Morton)..8 oz		300
Noodles & Butter Sauce (Penn. Dutch Brand)..........................1 cup		300
Ravioli, Cheese (Buitoni).......................4½ oz (about 12)		300
Spaghetti w Veal Frozen (Swanson RV Entree)....................................8¼ oz.		390
Lasagna w Meat Sauce (Buitoni)............1 pkg.		560
Noodles & Cheese Mic (Noodle Roni Parmesana) ....1 pkg.		650
Lasagna Mix (Stir-n-Serve)....................1 pkg.		700
Lasagna, Frozen (Celeste) 2 lg. ....1 pkg.		830

PASTRIES & TOASTER PASTRIES

Y I	Donut, Sugar-Sprice (Morton)................1	35
Donut, Cake (Hostess Family Carton) 1		140
Turnover, Apple (Pillsbury)....................1		150
Turnover, Blueberry (Pillsbury) 1		150
Turnover, Cherry (Pillsbury) 1		150
Toastettes, Apple (Nabisco)		190
Toastettes, Blueberry (Nabisco) 1		190
Toastettes, Brown Sugar Cinnamon 1		190
Toastettes, Cherry (Nabisco) 1		190
Toastettes, Peach (Nabisco) 1		190
Toastettes, Strawberry (Nabisco)...........1		190
Strudel, Pineapple-Cheese (Pepp. Farm)...............................one sixth 210		
Pop Tart, Chocolate Vanilla Creme (Kellogg's) 1		210
Pop Tart, Chocolate Fudge (Kellogg's) ...1		220
Strudel, Blueberry (Pepp. Farm) ....one sixth 240		
R	Dumpling, Apple (Pepp. Farm)................1	280
Pie Tart, Apple (Pepp. Farm)..................1		280
Pie, Tart, Blueberry (Pepp. Farm)...........1		280
Pie, Tart, Cherry (Pepp. Farm)................1		280
Dumpling, Peach (Pepp. Farm)...............1		290
Pie Tart, Chocolate (Pepp. Farm)...........1		310
Pie Tart Coconut Creme (Pepp. Farm)...1		310
Pie Tart, Lemon (Pepp. Farm).................1		320
Turnover, Apple (Pepp. Farm)..................1		320
Turnover, Blueberry (Pepp. Farm) 1		320
Turnover, Peach (Pepp. Farm) 1		320
Turnover, Strawberry (Pepp. Farm).........1		330
Turnover, Cherry (Pepp. Farm).................1		340
Turnover, Lemon (Pepp. Farm) 1		340
Turnover, Raspberry (Pepp. Farm) 1		340

    (G)=Green   (Y)=Yellow   (R)=Red

PIES, FROZEN

Strawberry Cream (Morton)....................1/6	165
Pumpkin (Morton) 20 0z............................1/6	170
Banana Cream (Morton).........................1/6	175
Lemon Cream (Morton)............................1/6	175
Neapolitan Cream (Morton) 1/6	180
Coconut Cream (Morton)..........................1/6	185
Cheesecake (Mrs. Smith's) 8" 1/6	205
Coconut Custard (Morton) 20 oz. 1/6	205
Banana Cream (Mrs. Smith's) 8" 1/6	215
Strawberry Cream (Mrs. Smith's) 8" 1/6	220
Lemon Cream (Mrs. Smith's) 1/6	225
Coconut Cream (Mrs. Smith) 8" 1/6	230
Blueberry (Morton) 20 oz. 1/6	240
Neapolitan Creme (Mrs. Smith's) 8" 1/6	240
Pumpkin (Mrs. Smith's) 8" 1/6	240
Chocolate Cream (Mrs. Smith's) 8".........1/6	245
Egg, Custard (Mrs. Smith's) 8" 1/6	245
Peach, (Morton) 20 oz. 1/6	245
Apple Tart (Mrs. Smith's) 8" 1/6	250
Cherry (Morton) 20 oz. 1/6	250
Mince (Morton) 20 oz. 1/6	250
Strawberry (Morton) 20 oz. 1/6	255
Lemon Meringue (Mrs. Smith's) 8" 1/6	260
Coconut Custard (Mrs. Smith's) 8" 1/6	265
Peach (Morton) 24 oz. 1/6	285
Blueberry (Mrs. Smith's) 8"....................1/6	290
Apple (Mrs. Smith's) 8" 295	
R Peach (Mrs. Smith's) 8" 1/6	300
Pineapple (Mrs. Smith's) 8" 1/6	300
Strawberry Shortcake, Nat. Juice	
(Mrs. Smith's) 9"...................................1/6	305
Apple, Dutch (Mrs. Smith's) 8" 1/6	310
Cherry (Mrs. Smith's) 8" 1/6	310
Raisin (Mrs. Smith's) 8" 1/6	315
Strawberry-Rhubard (Mrs. Smith's) 46 oz.1/6	315
Strawberry-Rhubard, Nat. Juice	
(Mrs. Smith's) 8"...................................1/6	320
Peach, Nat. Juice (Mrs. Smith's) 8" 1/6	330
Boston Cream (Mrs. Smith's) 8" 1/6	330
Mince (Mrs. Smith's) 8" 1/6	335
Apple Nat. Juice (Mrs. Smith's) 8".........1/6	340
Blueberry, Nat. Juice (Mrs. Smith's) 8" ..1/6	340
Cherry, Nat. Juice (Mrs. Smith's) 8" 1/6	340
Lemon (Mrs. Smith)s) 8" 1/6	340
Cherry (Morton) 24 oz...............................1/6	345
Pecan (Morton) 20 oz. 1/6	345
Lemon Krunch)mrs. Smith's) 8" 1/6	380
Cherry Shortcake, Nat. Juice....................1/6	
(Mrs. Smith's) 9"	390
Pecan (Mrs. Morton) 8" 1/6	430
Peach, Nat. Juice (Mrs. Smith's) 9" ...1/6	460
Blueberry, Nat. Juice (Mrs. Smith's) 9" ..1/6	480
Cherry, Nat. Juice (Mrs. Smith's) 9" 1/6	480
Peach (Morton) 46 oz. 1/6	535
Pineapple (Morton) 46 oz. 1/6	535
Cherry (Morton) 46 oz. 1/6	555
Strawberry Rhubarb (Mrs. Smith's) 46 oz.1/	580
Coconut Custard (Morton) 46 oz.............1/6	680
Mince (Morton) 46 oz. 1/6	700
Pecan (Morton) 46 oz. 1/6	765

PIES—SNACK

R Cherry (Hostess) 1	340

R	Apple (Hostess)...1	355
	Lemon (Hostess) 1	360

POULTY & GAME

Liver, Chicken, Simmered ....1 (about		40
	2"x2"x⅝"	
Chicken, Fried, Drumstick,		
w Bone(2½ lb. Fryer)...........................1		90
Chicken, Broiled, w/o skin ....2 oz.		120
Chicken, Fried, Thigh w		
Bone (2½ lb. Fryer).............................1		120
Chicken, Stewed, Light Meat		
w/o Skin..3oz.		150
Turkey, Roasted, Light Meat,		
Y w/o Skin..3 oz.		150
Chicken, Boned w Broth,		
Canned (Swanson)..............................3 oz.		155
Turkey, Boned w Broth,		
Canned (Swanson)..............................3 oz.		155
Chicken, Fried, Breast, w		
Bone (2½ lb. Fryer)..............................½		160
Chicken, Roasted, Dark Meat		
w/o Skin..3 oz.		160
Chicken, Roasted, Light Meat		
w/o Skin..3 oz.		160
Turkey, Roasted,Dark Meat		
w/o Skin..3 oz.		170
Chicken, Stewed, Dark Meat		
w/o Skin..3 oz.		180
Rabbit, Domesticated, Stewed ....3 oz.		180
Goose, Domesticated, Roasted...............3 oz.		200
Chicken Spread Canned (Swanson)........3 oz.		210
Chicken, Frozen, Fried (Swanson 6		
piece pkg.) ....3 oz.		335
Chicken, Frozen, Fried (Swanson		
12 piece pkg.) ....3 oz.		225
Liver, chicken, Simmered, Chopped ......1 cup		230
Liver, Chicken, Frozen (Swanson)..........1 pkg.		240
	(8 oz.)	
Chicken, Stewed, Light Meat		
w/o Skin, Diced....................................1 cup		250
Turkey, Roasted, Light Meat		
w/o Skin, Diced....................................1 cup		250
R chicken, Roasted, Dark Meat		
w/o Skin, Diced....................................1 cup		260
Chicken, Roasted, Light Meat w/o		
Skin, Diced...1 cup		260
Turkey, Roasted, Dark Meat		
w/o Skin, Diced....................................1 cup		280
Chicken, Stewed, Dark Meat		
w/o Skin, Diced....................................1 cup		290
Chicken, Spread, Canned		
(Underwood) ....1 can		300
	(4¾ oz)	
Turkey, Boneless, Canned....................1 cup		410
Turkey Salad (Spreadable) ....1 can		450
Chicken Salad, Canned (Spreadable) .....1 can		500

PUDDINGS

Chocolage, Mix (D Zerta) w		
whole milk ....½ cup		100
R	prep.	
Butterscotch, Mix (D-Zerta) w		
whole milk 5 oz. ....½ cup		110
	prep.	

(G)=Green   (Y)=Yellow   (R)=Red   213

Vanilla, Mix (D-Zerta) w whole milk	½ cup prep.	110
Indian, Canned (B&M)	½ cup	120
Lemon, Mix (Jell-O Whip 'n Chill) w whole milk	½ cup prep	135
Strawberry Mix (Jell-O Whip 'n Chill) w whole milk	½ cup prep.	135
Vanilla, Mix (Jell-O Whip 'n Chill) w whole milk	½ cup prep.	135
Chocolate Mix (Jel-O Whip 'n Chill) w whole milk	½ cup prep.	145
Tapioca (Minute Fluffy Pudding Recipe)	½ cup prep.	145
Custard Mix (Jell-O) w Whole Milk	½ cup prep.	165
Peach Mix (Jell-O Soft Swirl) w whole milk	½ cup prep.	170
Strawberry, Mix (Jell-O Soft Swirl) w whole milk	½ cup prep.	170
Tapioca, All Flavors, Mix (Jell-O)	½ cup prcp.	170
Banana Mix (Jell-O) w whole milk	½ cup prep.	175
R Choc Mix (Jell-O) w whole milk	½ cup prep.	175
Coconut Cream, Mix (Jell-O) w whole milk	½ cup prep.	175
Cool n Creamy, All Flavors, Frozen	½ cup	175
Vanilla Max (Jell-O) w whole milk	½ cup prep.	175
Banana, Canned (Del Monte)	5 oz.	180
Banana Mix (Jell-O Instant)	½ cup prep.	180
Butterscotch, Canned (Del Monte)	5 oz.	180
Butterscotch, Mix (Jell-O Instant)	½ cup prep.	180
Lemon, Mix (Jell-O)	½ cup prep.	180
Lemon, Mix (Jell-O Instant)	½ cup prep.	180
Vanilla, Mix (Jell-O Instant)	½ cup prep.	180
Choc., Canned (Del Monte)	½ cup.	190
Choc., Mix (Jell-O Instant)	½ cup prep.	190
Choc. Mix (Jell-O Soft Swirl) w whole milk	½ cup prep.	190
Choc. Fudge, Canned (Del Monte)	5 oz.	190
Coconut Cream Mix (Jell-O Instant) w whole milk	½ cup prep.	190
Vanilla, Canned (Del Monte)	5 oz.	190

RICE

R Spanish, Canned (Heinz)	1 can (7¼ oz.	150
White, Enriched, Instant, Cooked	1 cup hot	180
White, enriched, Parboiled, Long Grain, Cooked hot	1 cup	190
Spanish, Canned (Van Camp)	1 cup	190
White, Enriched, Cooked	1 cup hot	220
White, Unenriched, Cooked	1 cup hot	220
Brown, Long Grain	1 cup hot	230
Spanish, Frozen (Green Giant)	1 cup	230
White, Frozen w Peas & Mushrooms (Frn. Giant Medley)	1 cup	240
Pilaf, Frozen (Green Giant)	1 cup	250
R white and Wild, Frozen (Green Giant)	1 cup	250
Brown, Frozen in Beef Stock (Grn. Giant)	1 cup	250
White, Frozen w Peppers & Parsley (Grn. Giant Verdi)	1 cup	300
Rice and Peas, Frozen w Mushrooms (Bird's Eye Delux)	1 pkg.	345
Spanish Mix (Rice-A-Roni)	1 pkg.	720
Beef Flavor (Beef Rice-A-Roni)	1 pkg.	780
Chicken Flavor (Chicken Rice-A-Roni)	1 pkg.	800

ROLLS & BUNS

Rolls (Arnold's Party Tray)	1	40
Y Rolls, Pan, Round (Pepp. Farm Party)	1	45
Cinnamon Sticks, Frozen (Aunt Jemima)	1	50
Rolls, Dinner (Pillsbury Butterflake)	1	55
Rolls, (Arnold's Soft Tray)	1	60
Rolls, Butterfly (Pepp. Farm)	1	60
Rolls, Dinner, Parker House (Pillsbury)	1	60
Rolls, Old Fashioned (Pepp. Farm)	1	60
Rolls, Pan, Finger (Arnold's Family Egg Finger)	1	60
Rolls, Pan, Finger (Arnold's Finger Tray)	1	65
Rolls, Dinner (Pillsbury Snowflake)	1	70
Rolls, Pan (Pillsbury)	1	75
Rolls, Pan, Finger (Pepp. Farm Party)	1	75
Banana (Dromedary)	½" slice	75
Date (Dromedary)	½" slice	75
Rolls, Brown & Serve (Wonder)	1	80
Rolls, Dinner (Pepperidge Farm)	1	80
Rolls, Dinner, Parker House (Morton)	1	80
Orange, (Dromedary)	½" slice	80
Chocolate (Dromedary)	¼½" slice	85
Rolls, Dinner, Italian Crescent (Pillsbury)	1	90
R Rolls, Mix (Pillsbury)	1 prep	95
Rolls, Dinner, Crescent Pillsbury)	1	95
Cinnamon w Icing (Ballard)	1	105
Cinnamon Nut (Pepp. Farm)	1	110
Buns, Hamburger (Pepp. Farm)	1	115
Rolls, Dinner Crescent (Hungry Jack Buttermilk)	1	115
Cinnamon w Icing (Pillsbury)	1	115
Buns, Sandwich (Arnold's Soft)	1	120
Rolls, Club (Pepperidge Farm)	1	120
Buns, Frankfurter (Wonder)	1	125
Buns, Hamburger (Wonder)	1	125
Rolls, Golden Twist (Pepp. Farm)	1	130
Orange Danish (Pillsbury)	1	130
Rolls, Golden Twist (Pepp. Farm)	1	130
Orange Danish (Pillsbury)	1	130
Rolls, Dinner, Crescent (Pepp. Farm)	1	135
Cinnamon Danish w Raisins (Pillsbury)	1	135

Almond Danish (Pillsbury)	1	140
Cinnamon (Hungry Jack Butter Tastin')	1	145
Honey Buns (Morton)	1	145
Caramel Danish (Pillsbury)	1	155
Bagels, Egg	1	165
	(3″ diam.)	
Bagels, Water	1	165
	(3″ diam.)	

R	Buns, Frankfurter (Pepp. Farm)	1	165
	Rolls, (Arnold's Deli-Twist)	1	165
	Pecan Coffee Bun (Pepp. Farm)	1	190
	Cinnamon (Pillsbury Sweet 'n Simple)	1	240
	Orange (Pillsbury Sweet 'n Simple)	1	240
	Caramel (Pills. Sweet 'n Simple)	1	250
	Honey (Pills. Sweet 'n Simple)	1	250
	Rolls, French (Pepp. Farm Triple)	1	270
	Rolls, French (Pepp. Farm Twin)	1	390

SALAD DRESSINGS

	Italian (Good Seasons Low Galorie)	1 tbsp.	3
	Bleu Cheese (Slim-Ette Low Calorie)	1 tsp.	4
G	Thousand Island (Dia Mel)	1 tbsp.	4
	Green Golden (Slim-Ette Low Calorie)	1 tsp.	4
	French (Sweet 'n Low)	1 tbsp.	6
	Italian (Sween 'n Low)	1 tbsp.	6
	Bleu Cheese (Dieter's Gourmet Imitation)	1 tbsp.	12½
Y	Italian (Wish-Bone Low Calories)	1 tbsp.	15
	French (Wish-Bone Low Calorie)	1 tbsp.	25
	Russian (Wish-Bone Low Calorie)	1 tbsp.	25
	Thousand Island (Wish-Bone Low Calories)	1 tbsp.	25
	Russian (Wish-Bone)	1 tbsp.	55
	Salad Dressing (Hellmann's Spin-Blend)	1 tbsp.	55
	Tahitian Isle (Wish-Bone)	1 tbsp.	60
	French (Wish-Bone)	1 tbsp.	60
	Italian (Wish-Bone Rose)	1 tbsp.	60
	Garlic, French (Wish-Bone)	1 tbsp.	65
	Green Goddess (Wish-Bone)	1 tbsp.	70
	Thousand Island (Wish-Bone)	1 tbsp.	70
	Blue Cheese, Chunky (Whish-Bone)	1 tbsp.	75
	Garlic, Creamy (Wish-Bone)	1 tbsp.	75
	Italian, Wish-Bone	1 tbsp.	75
	Onion (Wish-Bone Calif.)	1 tbsp.	75
R	Thousand Island (Good Seasons Thick 'n Creamy)	1 tbsp.	80
	Cheese Garlic (Good Season)	1 tbsp.	85
	French (Good Seasons Old Fashion)	1 tbsp.	85
	Garlic (Good Seasons)	1 tbsp.	85
	Italian (Good Seasons)	1 tbsp.	85
	Blue Cheese (Good Seasons)	1 tbsp.	90
	Cheese Italian (Good Seasons)	1 tbsp.	90
	French (Good Seasons Riviera)	1 tbsp.	90
	Italian, Mild (Good Season)	1 tbsp.	90
	Italian (Good Seasons Thick 'n Creamy)	1 tbsp.	95
	Blue Cheese (Good Seasons Thick 'n Creamy)	1 tbsp.	100
	French (Good Seasons Thick 'n Creamy)	1 tbsp.	100

SAUCES & GRAVIES

Y	Gravy, Mix, Brown (Pillsbury)	½ cup	20
	Gravy, Mix, Home Style (Pillsbury)	½ cup	20

	Tomato (Contadina)	½ cup	40
	Tomato, Canned (Del Monte)	½ cup	40
	Swiss Steak (Contadina Cookbook)	½ cup	40
	Tomato w Mushrooms, Canned (Del Monte)	½ cup	50
	Tomato w Onion, Canned (Del Monte)	½ cup	50
	Gravy Mix, Chicken (Pillsbury)	½ cup	60
	Italian, Frozen (Celeste)	½ cup	70
	Pizza (Contadina)	½ cup	75
	Stroganoff (Contadina Cookbook)	½ cup	80
	Meat Loaf (Contadina Cookbook)	½ cup	85
	Mushroom (Contadina Cookbook)	½ cup	100
	Spaghetti (Ragu)	5 oz.	105
R	Spaghetti w Mushrooms (Ragu)	5 oz.	105
	Spaghetti w Clams (Ragu)	5 oz.	110
	Spaghetti w Meat (Ragu)	5 oz.	115
	Chili, Canned (Stokely-Van Camp)	½ cup	120
	Marinara, Ragu	5 oz.	120
	Pizza (Ragu)	5 oz.	120
	Spaghetti, Pepperoni Flavored (Ragu)	5 oz.	120
	Tomato Catsup (Del Monte)	½ cup	120
	Seafood Cocktail (Del Monte)	½ cup	140
	Sweet 'n Sour (Contadina Cookbook)	½ cup	160
	Barbecue (Open Pit)	½ cup	210
	Barbecue (Open Pit Hickory Smoke Flavor)	½ cup	220
	Barbecue (Open Pit Hot 'n Spicy)	½ cup	220
	Barbecue w Onions (Open Pit)	½ cup	220

SNACK FOODS

Y	Popcorn, Popped, Plain, Large Kernel	1 cup	25
	Popcorn, Popped, w Oil and Salt Large Kernel	1 cup	40
	Dehydrated Apple Snack (Weight Watchers)	1 pkg.	50
	Potato Chips (Pringles)	1 pkg.	50
	Potato Chips (Pringles)	10	75
	Chipsters, Potato Snacks	1 oz.	130
	Onion Rings (Wonder)	1 oz.	135
	Bacon Rinds (Wonder)	1 oz.	145
	Soy Beans, Roasted (Soy Ahoy)	1 oz.	145
	Soy Beans, Roasted (Soy Town)	1 oz.	145
R	Soy Beans, Roasted, Unsalted (Soy Ahoy)	1 oz.	145
	Soy Beans, Roasted, Unsalted (Soy Town)	1 oz	145
	Taco Tortilla Chips (Wonder)	1 oz.	145
	Tortilla Chips (Wonder)	1 oz.	150
	Cheese Twists (Wonder)	1 oz.	155
	Potato Chips, Barbecue (Wonder)	1 oz.	155
	Corn Capers (Wonder)	1 oz.	160
	Potato Chips (Wonder)	1 oz.	160
	Corn Chips (Wonder)	1 oz.	165
	Pretzels (Mister Salty Very-Thin)	10	200

SOFT DRINKS

	Club Soda (Santiba)	8 fl. oz.	0
	Club Soda (Schweppes)	8 fl. oz.	0
	Club Soda (Shasta)	8 fl. oz.	0
G	Club Soda (Canada Dry)	8 fl. oz.	0-1
	Cola (Diet Rite)	8 fl. oz.	0-1
	Cola (Diet Pepsi)	8 fl. oz.	0-1
	Tab	8 fl. oz.	0-1
	Cola (Canada Dry Diet)	8 fl. oz.	1

(G)=Green (Y)=Yellow (R)=Red 215

	Creme Soda (Canada Dry Diet)	8 fl. oz.	1
	Orange (Canada Dry Diet)	8 fl. oz.	1
	Orange (Diet Rite)	8 fl. oz.	1
	Pink Grapefruit (Canada Dry Diet)	8 fl. oz.	1
	Root Beer (Canada Dry Diet)	8 fl. oz.	1
G	Strawberry (Canada Dry Diet)	8 fl. oz.	1
	Black Cherry (Canada Dry Diet)	8 fl. oz.	2
	Coffee (Canada Dry Diet)	8 fl. oz.	2
	Fresca	8 fl. oz.	2
	Lemon (Canada Dry Diet)	8 fl. oz.	2
	Lemon-Lime (Diet Rite)	8 fl. oz.	2
	Ginger Ale (Canada Dry Diet)	8 fl. oz.	3
	Ginger Ale (Fanta)	8 fl. oz.	80
	Mixer Collins (Canada Dry)	8 fl. oz.	84
	Tonic Water (Santiba)	8 fl. oz.	84
	Ginger Ale (Santiba)	8 fl. oz.	84
	Ginger Ale (Canada Dry)	8 fl. oz.	85
	Mixer Sour (Canada Dry)	8 fl. oz.	90
	Mixer Whiskey Sour (Canada Dry)	8 fl. oz.	90
	Tonic Water (Canada Dry)	8 fl. oz.	90
	Tonic Water (Schweppes)	8 fl. oz.	90
	Ginger Beer (Schweppes)	8 fl. oz.	95
	Lemon (Canada Dry Hi-Spot)	8 fl. oz.	95
	Cola (Coca-Cola)	8 fl. oz.	96
	Mr. Piff	8 fl. oz.	96
	Simba	8 fl. oz.	96
	Sprite	8 fl. oz.	96
	Birch Beer (Canada Dry)	8 fl. oz.	100
	Bitter Lemon (Canada Dry)	8 fl. oz.	100
	Cola (RC with a twist)	8 fl. oz.	100
	Half and Half (Canada Dry)	8 fl. oz.	100
	Jamaica Cola (Canada Dry)	8 fl. oz.	100
	Root Beer (Canada Dry Root)	8 fl. oz.	100
	Teem	8 fl. oz.	100
	Root Beer (Fanta)	8 fl. oz.	100
	Cola (Pepsi Cola)	8 fl. oz.	105
	Cola (Royal Crown)	8 fl. oz.	105
R	Grapfruit (Shasta)	8 fl. oz.	105
	Upper 10	8 fl. oz.	105
	Wink	8 fl. oz.	105
	Root Beer (Patio)	8 fl. oz.	110
	Grape (Fanta)	8 fl. oz.	112
	Creme Soda (Shasta)	8 fl. oz.	115
	Root Beer (Shasta)	8 fl. oz.	115
	Tiki (Shasta)	8 fl. oz.	115
	Island Mixer (Santiba)	8 fl. oz.	115
	Blk. Cherry (Shasta)	8 fl. oz.	120
	Cactus Cooler (Canada Dry)	8 fl. oz.	120
	Grape (Shasta)	8 fl. oz.	120
	Orange (Fanta)	8 fl. oz.	120
	Purple Passion (Canada Dry)	8 fl. oz.	120
	Strawberry (Canada Dry California)	8 fl. oz.	120
	Wild Raspberry (Shasta)	8 fl. oz.	120
	Grape (Niki)	8 fl. oz.	125
	Mountain Dew	8 fl. oz.	125
	Orange (Canada Dry)	8 fl. oz.	125
	Root Ber (Niki)	8 fl. oz.	125
	Bitter lemon (Schweppes)	8 fl. oz.	130
	Cream Soda (Canada Dry)	8 fl. oz.	130
	Fruit Punch (Niki)	8 fl. oz.	130
	Ginger Ale (Shast)	8 fl. oz.	130
	Grape (Canada Dry)	8 fl. oz.	130
	Grape (Patio)	8 fl. oz.	130
	Mixer Collins (Shasta)	8 fl. oz.	130
	Mixer Sour (Shasta)	8 fl. oz.	130
	Mixer, Vodka (Shasta)	8 fl. oz.	130

	Orange (Patio)	8 fl. oz.	130
	Orange (Shasta)	8 fl. oz.	130
	Tahitian Treat (Canada Dry)	8 fl. oz.	130
	Wild Cherry (Canada Dry)	8 fl. oz.	135
R	Orange (Nehi)	8 fl. oz.	135
	Lemon-Lime (Shasta)	8 fl. oz.	150
	Cherry Cola (Shasta)	8 fl. oz.	160
	Cola (Shasta)	8 fl. oz.	160
	Strawberry (Shasta)	8 fl. oz.	160

SOUPS

G	Onion Broth (Weight Watchers	1 pkt	7
	Beef-Flavored (Lipton Cup-A-Broth)	1 env. (6 fl. oz)	20
	Broth, Beef (Swanson)	10 oz.	25
	Chicken-Flavored (Lipton Cup-A-Broth)	1 env. (6 fl. oz)	25
	Onion (Lipton Cup-A-Soup	1 env. (6 fl. oz)	30
	Turkey Noodle (Campbells's Low Sodium)	½ can	30
	Broth, Beef (Campbell's)	10 oz. prep	35
	Noodle w Beef Flavor (Lipton Cup-A-Soup)	1 env. (6 fl. oz.)	35
	Onion (Lipton)	1 cup	35
	Broth, Chicken (Swanson)	10 oz.	40
	Consomme (Campbell's)	10 oz.	40.
	Mushroom w Beef Flavor (Lipton)	1 cup	40
	Noodle, Chicken Flavor (Lipton Cup-A-Soup)	1 env. (6 fl. oz.)	40
	Vegetable Campbells's Low Sodium)	½ can	40
Y	Vegetable Beef (Campbell's Low Sodium)	½ can	40
	Noodle w chicken meat (Lipton cup-A-Soup)	1 env. (6 fl. oz.)	45
	Vegetable (Lipton Cup-A-Soup)	1 env. (6 fl. oz.)	45
	Broth, Chicken (Campbell's)	10 oz. prep.	50
	Tomato (Campbell's Low Sodim)	½ can	50
	Noodle w Chicken broth (Lipton)	1 cup	55
	Noodle w chicken broth (Ring-O-Noodle Lipton)	1 cup	60
	Turkey Noodle (Lipton	1 cup	60
	Vegetable Beef (Lipton)	1 cup	60
	Chicken Rice (Lipton)	1 cup	65
	Mushroom, Cream of (Campbell's Low Sodium)	½ can	65
	Noodle (Beef Flavor w Vegetables (Lipton)	½ cup	65
	chicken Gumbo (Cambell's)	10 oz. prep.	70
	Green Pea (Campbell's Low Sodim)	½ can	70
	Noodle w Diced Chicken (Lipton)	1 cup	70
	Tomato Vegetable w Noodles (Lipton)	1 cup	70

Food	Serving	Value
Noodle w Chicken Broth (Lipton Giggle Noodle)	1 cup	75
Vegetable w Noodles (Lipton)	1 cup	75
Chicken Rice (Campbell's)	10 oz. prep.	80
Chicken and Stars (Campbell's)	10 oz. prep.	80
Onion (Campbell's)	10 oz. prep.	80
Oyster Stew (Campbell's)	10 z. prep.	80
Tomato (Lipton Cup-A-Soup)	1 env. (6 fl. oz.)	80
Beef Noodle (Campbell's)	10 oz. prep.	90
Chicken Noodle (Campbell's)	10 oz. prep.	90
Chicken Noodle (Campbell's Noodle O's)	10 oz. prep.	90
Y Chicken Vegetable (Campbell's)	10 oz. prep	90
Mushroom, Cream of (Lipton Cup-A-Soup)	1 env. (6 fl. oz.)	90
Potato, Cream of (Campbell's)	10 oz. prep.	90
Turkey Noodle (Campbell's)	10 oz. prep.	90
Turkey Vegetable (Campbells)	10 oz. prep.	90
Vegetable Beef (Campbell's)	10 oz. prep.	90
Vegetable w Noodles (Campbell's Noodle-O's)	10 oz. prep.	90
Vegetable, Old Fashioned (Campbell's)	10 oz. prep.	90
Vegetarian Vegetable (Campbell's)	10 oz. prep.	90
Vegetarian Vegetable (Heinz Great American)	½ can	90
Chicken, Cream of (Lipton Cup-A-Soup)	1 env. (6 fl. oz.)	95
Asparagus, Cream of (Campbell's)	10 oz. prep.	100
Beef, (Campbell's)	10 oz. prep.	100
Broth, Sctoch (Campbell's)	10 oz. prep.	100
Clam Chowder, Manhattan Style (Campbell's)	10 oz. prep	100
R Clam Chowder, New England (Campbell's)	10 oz. prep.	100
Mushroom Golden (Campbell's)	10 oz. prep.	100
Noodle w chicken (Campbell's Curly Noodle)	10 oz. prep.	100
Potato (Lipton)	1 cup	100
Vegetable (Campbell's)	10 oz. prep.	100
Minestrone (Campbell's)	10 oz. prep.	110
Celery Cream of 'Campbell's)	10 oz. prep.	110
Noodle and Ground Beef (Campbell's)	10 oz. prep.	110
Tomato (Campbell's)	10 oz. prep.	110
Chicken 'n Dumplings (Campbell's)	10 oz. prep.	120
Shrimp Cream of (Campbell's)	10 oz. prep.	120
Stock Pot (Campbell's)	10 oz. prep.	120
Bean Black (Campbell's)	10 oz. prep.	130
Green Pea (Lip Cup-A-Soup)	1 env. (6 fl. oz.)	130
Pepper Pot (Campbell's)	10 oz. prep.	130
Chicken Cream of (Campbell's)	10 oz. prep	140
Green Pea (Lipton)	1 cup	140
Potato Cream of Made w Water & Milk (Campbell's)	10 oz. prep.	140
Tomato (Heinz Great American)	½ can	140
Tomato Rice (Cambell's)	10 oz.	140
Vegetable (Campbell's Chunky)	½ can	140
Mushroom Cream of (Campbell's)	10 oz. prep.	150
R Tomato Bisque (Campbell's)	10 oz. prep.	150
Chicken w Rice (Campbell's Chunky)	½ can	160
Clam Chowder (Campbell's Chunky)	½ can	160
Tomato-Beef Noodle-O's (Campbell's)	10 oz. prep.	160
Turkey (Campbell's Chunky)	½ can	160
Oyster Stew Made w Milk (Campbell's)	10 oz. prep.	170
Cheddar Cheese (Campbell's)	10 oz. prep.	180
Green Pea (Campbell's)	10 oz. prep.	180
Chili Beef (Campbell's)		190
Clam Chowder New England, made w Milk (Campbell's)	10 oz. prep	190
Bean w Bacon (Campbell's)	10 oz. prep.	200
Chicken (Campbell's Chunky)	4 can	200
Beef (Campbell's Chunky)	½ can	210
Hot Dog Bean (Campbell's)	10 oz. prep.	210
Shrimp Cream of made w Milk (Campbell's)	10 oz. prep.	210
Sirloin Burger (Campbell's chunky)	½ can	210

R	Split Pea w Ham (Campbell's) ....10 oz. prep.	210
	Split Pea w Ham (Campbell's Chunky)................................½ can	220

TEA

G	Instant, Lemon Flavored (Lipton) ....8 fl. oz.	3
	Iced Mix, Lemon Flavored (Lipton Low Calorie)............................8 fl. oz.	5
R	Iced Mix, Lemon Flavored (Lipton).........8 fl. oz.	105
	Iced in a Can (Lipton) ....8 fl. oz.	140

TOPPINGS

G	Flavoring (No Cal. all flavors) ....1 tbsp.	1
	Pancake & Waffle Topping (No Cal) ......1 tbsp	1
	Blackberry Jam (Dia Mel Imitation)........1 tbsp	6
Y	Strawberry Preserves (Dia Mel Imitation) ....1 tbsp	6
	Chocolate Topping (Low Cal)..................1 tbsp.	8
	Orange Marmelade (TYillie Lew Imitation)......................................1 tbsp.	12
	Topping, Non-dairy (Cool Whip) ....2 tbsp.	32
	Chocolate Flavored (Hershey's)..............2 tbsp.	70
	Fudge (Hershey's) ....2 tbsp.	100
	Chocolate Flavored (Bosco)....................2 tbsp.	110
	Topping Mix (Dream Whip) ....½ c prep.	115
R	Strawberry (Smucker's) ....2 tbsp.	120
	Cherry (Smucker's) ....2 tbsp.	130
	Chocolate Flavored (Smucker's).............2 tbsp.	130
	Fudge (Smucker's) ....2 tbsp.	130
	Pineapple (Smucker's)..............................2 tbsp.	130
	Butterscotch Flavor (Smucker's) ....2 tbsp.	140
	Caramel Flavor (Smucker's) ....2 tbsp.	140
	chocolate (Smucker's Swiss Milk)..2 tbsp.	140
	Fudge, Chocolate-Mint (Smucker's)...2 tbsp.	140
	Peanut Butter Caramel (Smucker's)...2 tbsp.	150
	Pecans in Syrup (Smucker's)...................2 tbsp	150
	Walnuts in Syrup (Smucker's) ....2 tbsp	150

VEGETABLES

G	Lettuce, Boston or Bibb (5" diam. head)..1 lg. leaf 2 med of 3 small	2
	Parsley, Raw, chopped.............................1 tbsp.	2
	Onions, Raw, Chopped ....1 tbsp.	4
	Celery, Green, Raw (8" x 1½" at root end)...1	8
	Lettuce, Iceberg, Shredded or chopped ....1 cup	8
	Watercress, Raw, Whole...........................1 cup about 10 springs	8
	Asparagus, Green, Fresh, Cooked, Drained, Spears ....4 spears (½" diam at base)	10

	Cabbage, Chinese, Raw, Shredded Coarsley ....1 cup	10
	Carrots, Raw in strips (¼"x2½-3")...6-8 (1 oz)	10
	Endive Curly, Raw, Cut.............................1 cup	10
	Lettuce, Iceberg, chunks, Small..............1 cup	10
	Lettuce, loose leaf or bunching, chopped or shredded.............................1 cup	10
	Radishes, Raw, Red..................................10 med.	10
	Onions, Raw, Green..................................2 med or 6 small	14
	Spinach, Raw, chopped............................1 cup	14
	Mushrooms, Canned (Green Giant).........2 oz	15
	Peppers, Green, Sweet, Raw ....1 (about 5/lb)	16
	Cabbage, Raw, Shredded Coarsely.........1 cup	18
	Celery, Green, Raw, Diced or chopped..1 cup	20
	Cucumbers, Raw, Pared, Sliced (⅛" thick)....................................1 cup	20
	Mushrooms, Raw, Sliced, Chopped or Diced ....1 cup	20
	Cabbage, Raw, Red, Shredded Coarsely...1 cup	22
	Beet Greens, Fresh, Leave and Stems, Cooked, Drained ....1 cup	25
	Peppers, Green, Sweet, Sliced Cooked, Drained ....1 cup	25
	Pepers, Red, Sweet, Raw ....1 (about 5/lb)	25
G	Watercress, Raw, Chopped Finely ....1 cup	25
	Asparagus, Green, Fresh, Cooked, Drained, Pieces ....1 cup	30
	Beet Greens, Fresh, Leaves & Stems Cooked & Drained.................................1 cup	25
	Cauliflower, Raw, Sliced, Flowerbuds..1 cup	25
	Beans, Green, Fresh, Cookes, Drained...1 cup	30
	Beans, Wax, Fresh, Cooked, Drained...1 cup	30
	Beets, Fresh, Whole, Cooked, Drained...2 beets (2" diam)	30
	Cabbage, Fresh, Cooked, Drained...........1 cup	30
	Cauliflower, Fresh, Cooked, Drained, Flowerbuds.............................1 cup	30
	Chard, Swiss, Fresh, Leaves Cooked, Drained ....1 cup	30
	Cress, Garden, Cooked, Drained ....1 cup	30
	Mustard Greens, Fresh Cooked, Drained ....1 cup	30
	Squash, Summer, Cooked, Drained, Diced....................................1 cup	30
	Turnip Greens, Cooked, Drained...1 cup	30
	Asparagus, Green, Canned (Del Monte)...1 cup	35
	Asparagus, Canned, White & Green Tipped (Del Monte)....................1 up	35
	Beans, Green, Canned, Whole (Del Monte)..................................1 cup	35
	Beans, Wax, Canned, (Del Monte) ....1 cup	35

Food	Measure	Value
Beans, Wax, Canned, French (Del Monte)	1 cup	35
Bean Sprouts, Raw	1 cup	35
Bean Sprouts, Cooked Drained	1 cup	35
Dandelion Greens, Cooked Drained	1 cup (not pressed down)	35
Mushrooms, Frozen in Butter Sauce (Green Giant)	2 oz	35
Turnips, Cooked, Cubed, Drained	1 cup	35
Asparagus, Canned (Green Giant)	1 cup	40
Asparagus, Canned (Le Sueur)	1 cup	40
Asparagus, Canned (Stokely-Van Camp)	1 cup	40
Asparagus, Frozen, Cut (Bird's Eye 5 minute)	1 cup	40
Beans, Green, Canned, Cut (Del Monte)	1 cup	40
Beans, Green, Canned, Tiny, Whole (Del Monte)	1 cup	40
Beans, Green, Canned (Green Giant)	1 cup	40
Beans, Green, Canned (Stokely-Van Camp)	1 cup	40
Beans, Green, Canned, French (Del Monte)	1 cup	40
Beans, Green, Canned, Seasoned (Del Monte)	1 cup	40
Beans, Wax, Canned, (Green Giant)	1 cup	40
G Beans, Wax, Canned (Libby's)	1 cup	40
G Broccoli Fresh, Cut (½" pieces) Cooked, Drained	1 cup	40
Eggplant, Fresh, Diced, Cooked, Drained	1 cup	40
Mustard Greens, Frozen (Bird's Eye)	1 cup	40
Onions, Frozen, Chopped (Ore-Ida)	1 cup	40
Sauerkraut, Canned (Stokely-Van Camp)	1 cup	40
Spinach, Cooked, Drained	1 cup	40
Spinach, Canned (Stokely-Van Camp)	1 cup	40
Squash, Summer Frozen (Bird's Eye 5-minute)	1 cup	40
Turnip Greens, Canned (Stokely-Van Camp)	1 cup	40
Zucchini, 1 cup Forzen (Brid's Eye 5-minute)	pkg.	40
Artichoke Hearts, Frozen (Brid's Eye Deluxe)	5-6	45
Asparagus, Frozen Spears (Bird's Eye 5-minute)	pkg.	45
Beans, Green, Frozen, Cut (Bird's Eye 5-minute)	2/3 pk.	45
Beans, Green, Frozen, Cut (Brid's Eye De-luxe)	2/3 pkg.	45
Beans, Italian, Frozen (Birds Eye 5-Min.)	pkg.	45
Beans, Green, Frozen, French Style (Bird's Eye-5 min)	pkg.	45
Beans, Wax, Canned (Stokely Van Camp)	1 cup	45
Broccoli, Fresh, Stalks, whole, Cooked, Drained	1 med.	45
Carrots, Raw, Grated or Shredded	1 cup	45
Cauliflower, Frozen (Bird's Eye 5-Min.)	pkg.	45
Kale, Leaves, w/o stems, Cooked, Drained	1 cup	45
Okra, Fresh, Sliced, Cooked, Drained	1 cup	45
Onions, Raw, sliced	1 cup	45
Sauerkraut, Canned (Libby's)	1 cup	45
Spinach, Canned (Libby's)	1 cup	45
Spinach, Canned (Del Monte)	1 cup	45
Spinach, Canned (Libby's)	1 cup	45
Tomatoes, Caned, Whole (Stokely-Van Camp)	1 cup	45
Turnip Greens, Frozen (Bird's Eye)	1 cup	45
Beans, Wax, Frozen (Bird's Eye 5-Min.)	pkg.	50
Beets, Canned, Shoestring (Libby's)	1 cup	50
Broccoli, Frozen, Spears, Baby (Bird's Eye Deluxe)	2/3 pkg.	50
Carrots, Fresh, Cooked, Sliced, Drained	1 cup	50
Sauerdraut, Canned (Del Monte)	1 cup	50
Soy Beans, Sprouted Seeds, Raw	1 cup	50
Soy Beans, Sprouted Seeds, Cooked, Drained	1 cup	50
G Spinach, Frozen, Chopped (Bird's Eye 5-Min.)	2/3 pkg.	50
Tomatoes, Canned, Whole, Peeled (Del Monte)	1 cup	50
Tomatoes, Raw, Unpeeled	1 (4" diam.)	50
Beans, Green, Frozen, French w mushrooms (Bird's Eye Deluxe)	2/3 pkg.	55
Brocolli, Frozen, Chopped (Bird's Eye 5-Min)	2/3 pkg.	55
Broccoli, Frozen, Spears (Bird's Eye 5 Min)	2/3 pkg.	55
Okra, Frozen, Whole (Bird's Eye)	1 cup	55
Tomatoes, Canned (Contadina)	1 cup	60
Beets, Fresh, Diced or Sliced	1 cup	60
Brussels Sprouts, Fresh (1¼"x1½"-7-8)	1 cup	60
Carrots, Canned, (Del Monte)	1 cup	60
Carrots, Canned (Le Sueur)	1 cup	60
Carrots, Canned (Sliced S&W)	1 cup	60
Collards, Fresh, Cooked, Drained	1 cup	60
Collard Greens, Frozen (Bird's Eye)	pkg.	60
Kale, Frozen (Bird's Eye)	1 cup	60
Pimientos, Canned (Stokely-Van Camp)	1 cup	60
Potatoes, Frozen, Fried (Ore-Ida Golden Crinkles)	10	60
Potatoes, Frozen, Fried (Ore-Ida Golden Fries)	10	60
Rutabaha, Fresh, Cooked, Drained, Cubed or Sliced	1 cup	60
Tomatoes, Cooked	1 cup	60
Tomatoes, Canned, Wedges (Del Monte)	1 cup	60

Zucchini, Canned, in Tomato
  Sauce (Del Monte) ....1 cup 60
Beet, Canned (Libby's) ....1 cup 65
Carrots, Canned (Stokely-
  Van Camp) ....1 cup 65
Brussels Sprouts, Frozen, Baby
  (Bird's Eye Delux) ....1 cup 70
Corn, Fresh, Cooked............1 (5" x 70
Mixed, San Francisco Style 1½-¾")
  (Green Giant)............1 cup 70
Okra, Frozen, Cut (Bird's Eye) ....1 cup 70
Potatoes, Boiled, After peeling ....1 med. (2- 70
  ½" diam)

G Tomatoes, Canned, Stewed
  (Del Monte) ....1 cup 70
Tomatoes, Canned, Sliced
  (Contadina) ....1 cup 75
Tomatoes, Canned, Stewed
  (Contadina) ....1 cup 75
Beans, Green, Frozen, French
  in Butter Sauce (Frn Giant) ....1 C 80
Beans, Green, Frozen w Onions &
  Bacon in Sauce (Grn Giant) ....1 cup 80
Mixed, Canned (Del Monte)............1 cup 80
Pumpkin, Canned (Del Monte)............1 cup 80
Pumpkin, Canned (Libby's) ....1 cup 80
Pumpkin, Canned (Stokely-
  Van Camp) :............1 cup 80
Potatoes, Frozen, Fried (Ore-Ida
  Cottage Fries) 10 85
Potatoes, Canned (Del Monte)............1 cup 90

Y Spinach, Frozen in Butter Sauce
  (Green Giant)............1 cup 90
Tomatoes, Canned, Diced in
  Puree (Contadian) ....1 cup 90
Broccoli, Frozen in Butter
  Sauce (Green Giant)............1 cup 100
Mixed, Frozen (Bird's Eye 5 Min.)............1 cup 100
Onions, Frozen Whole
  (Bird's Eye)............1 cup 100

R Parsnips, Diced, Cooked,
  Drained............1 cup 100
Peas, Canned, Sweet, Tiny
  (Del Monte) ....1 cup 100
Peas, Canned, and Carrots
  (Del Monte)............1 cup 100
Peas and Carrots, Canned
  (Libby's)............1 cup 100

Potatoes, Boiled in Skin............1 med. 100
  2½" diam)
Potatoes, Canned (Stokely-
  Van Camp) ....1 cup 100
Tomatoe Puree (Contadina) ....1 cup 100
Beans, Green, Frozen, French w
  Almonds (Bird's Eye Deluxe)............1 cup 110
Beans, Green, Frozen w
  Mushroom Sauce (Grn Giant) ....1 cup 110
Beets, Frozen, w Orange Flavor
  Flavor Glaze (Bird's Eye De-luxe)........pkg. 110
Carrots, Frozen in Butter
  Sauce (Grn Giant) ....1 cup 110
Onions, Frozen in Cream
  Sauce (Grn Giant) ....1 cup 110
Peas, Fresh, Cooked, Drained............1 cup 110
Peas, Canned, Early (Del
  Monte)............1 cup 110
Peas, Frozen, and Carrots
  (Bird's Eye 5-min.) ....1 cup 110
Peas, Frozen w Celery
  (Bird's Eye Deluxe) ....1 cup 110
Potatoes, Hash Brown (Ore-
R Ida Shredded Hash Browns)............1 cup 110
Peas, Canned (Libby's)............1 cup 115
Beans, Italian, Frozen in
  Tomato Sauce (Grn Giant) ....1 cup 120
Brussels Sprouts, Frozen, in
  Butter Sauce (Grn Giant) ....1 cup 120
Mixed, Florida Style (Grn Giant)............1 cup 120
Peas, Caned, Seasoned
  (Del Monte) ....1 cup 120
Spinach, Frozen, Creamed
  (Bird's Eye De-luxe) ....pkg. 120
Tomato Salad, Canned,
  Jellied (Contadina)............1 cup 120
Beans, Green, Frozen in
  Mushroom Sauce (Grn Giant) ....1 cup 130
Mixed, Frozen in Butter
  Sauce (Grn Giant) ....1 cup 130
Mixed, Chinese Style Frozen
  (Bird's Eye) ....1 cup 130
Peas, Canned (Grn Giant)............1 cup 130
Peas, Canned (Le Sueur)............1 cup 130
Peas, Canned, Honey Pod
  (Stokely-Van Camp)............1 cup 130
Peas, Canned, w Onions
  (Grn Giant) ....1 cup 130

These new books can

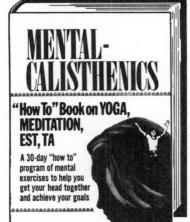

MENTAL CALISTHENICS

Here's an exciting book that offers you a 30 day How-To Program of mental exercises that combine the techniques of meditation, yoga, psychoanalysis, primal, transactional analysis, written in swift-reading language. Steven West, the well known psychologist and author gives you step-by-step instruction in this easy-to-read book.   **$9.95**

- **Learn How To Use The Alpha Dimension**
- **Understanding Your Strengths And Weakness**
- **Learn How To Use Body Language**
- **Understand How To Change Your Programming**
- **Learn How To Eliminate Bad Habits Easily**
- **Understand How To Approach Sex Positively**

BONUS: Long Playing Record That Teaches You How To Use The Alpha Dimension.

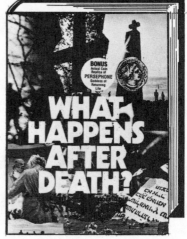

WHAT HAPPENS AFTER DEATH?
You Don't Have To Die To Find Out

Now, for the first time, you can learn the entire truth about Life and Death. Here, in one easy-to-read volume you will find the answers to many of the questions that have puzzled and frightened you over the years. Here is a book that will enlighten you and comfort you more than any book you have ever read
                                                    $9.95
- **Truth About The Origin Of Man**
- **New Evidence About Reincarnation**
- **Cases Of People Dying And Returning**
- **Out-Of-Body Experience Reports**
- **Mythology, Magic and Religion**
- **Visitors From Outer Space/UFOS**
- **Mysterious World Of Dreams**

BONUS: Actual Coin Replica of PERSEPHONE The Goddess Of Returning Life

---

Your tape player can become a learning machine

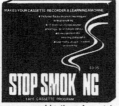

HOW TO STOP SMOKING IN 30 DAYS
Here's a complete, step-by-step program on a cassette that you can play on your cassette player and learn how to stop smoking swiftly, simply, easily. This new program uses a combination of mental exercises, meditation and behavior modification that will release you from your smoking habit in 30 days time!   **$9.95**

- **You'll Feel Better, Look Better, Live Longer!**
- **You Will Not Gain Weight With This Program!**
- **Your Smoker's Cough Will Disappear Forever!**
- **You Won't Feel Frustrated Or Strung Out!**
- **You'll Breathe Easier, Sleep Better!**

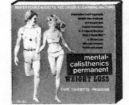

NEW PERMANENT WEIGHT LOSS PROGRAM
Now, for the first time, here's a program that you can play on your cassette player that will teach you how to lose weight easily, swiftly, permanently! Steven West, a leading psychologist and author combines the techniques of meditation, psychology and nutrition in a new, permanent, weight loss program that you can use immediately.   **$9.95**

- **Quick Results With Weight Loss Of 3 to 4 Pounds Each Week You Continue This Program!**
- **This Is An Easy Program — No Complicated Calorie Counting Or Expensive Time Consuming Gadgets!**
- **Improve Your Health At The Same Time You Begin To Look Better, Feel Bettery Day By Day!**
- **Gain New Energy, New Relaxation, Find A New Zest For Life And A Better Outlook On Life!**

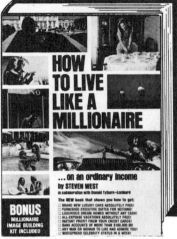
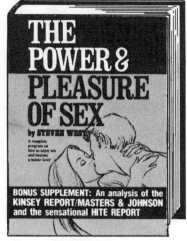